ALSO BY THOMAS J. MOORE

HEART FAILURE

THOMAS J. MOORE

SIMON & SCHUSTER

LIFESPAN

WHO LIVES LONGER
—AND WHY

NEW YORK LONDON TORONTO SYDNEY TOKYO SINGAPORE

SIMON & SCHUSTER
Simon & Schuster Building
Rockefeller Center
1230 Avenue of the Americas
New York, New York 10020

Designed by Karolina Harris
Manufactured in the United States of America
1 3 5 7 9 10 8 6 4 2
Library of Congress Cataloging-in-Publication Data
Moore, Thomas J., date.
Lifespan : who lives longer—and why / Thomas J. Moore.
p.   cm.
Includes bibliographical references and index.
1. Longevity.   2. Health risk assessment.   3. Communicable diseases.   4. Virus
diseases.   I. Title.
QP85.M55   1993
612.6'8—dc20   92-40669 CIP
ISBN 0-671-72966-7

Chapter 9 was previously published in *Washingtonian* magazine in modified form.

IN MEMORY OF JANE KAUFFMAN MOORE

CONTENTS

AUTHOR'S NOTE

This book is written in a narrative style that emphasizes readability over scholarly documentation. However, a separate section (at the end) provides detailed citations as well as suggestions for further reading.

—TJM
Center for Health Policy Research
George Washington University
Washington, D.C., 1992

BOOK

1

LONGEVITY GAINS

CHAPTER ONE

DIMENSIONS OF THE OLDEST

DREAM

The desire for a lifespan that is longer than nature ordinarily provides may be as unique and universal a human trait as the marvel of language. For uncounted thousands of years, humans in a state of nature survived about 15 to 17 years on the average. One might define human progress as a relentless assault on that outcome, an effort that has increased the average lifespan today in the most advanced countries to almost 80 years. The greatest catastrophes in human history can be measured in their impact on life expectancy—some unfortunate populations have seen their typical lifespan reduced almost to zero. Also, it may be that the achievements of a just society may be more reliably measured in the longevity and health of its citizens than in the beauty of its art, the might of its armies, or the economic riches it has acquired.

In many cultures, thoughtful men and women have enumerated values they described as more important than a life of maximum possible length. These include religious faith, defense of country, family, comrades and personal honor. Repeatedly, individuals have enshrined these values through the sacrifice of their own lives. Nevertheless, it is a long life itself that provides the standard against which all other major values are judged.

Longevity has also become an important daily or weekly preoccupation of millions of people around the world. The common commandments for daily living once sprang from moral or religious authorities. Today they involve precepts alleged to promote a longer lifespan, and are issued by medical authorities. Modern commandments involve exercise; not smoking; wearing seat belts; getting immunizations; avoiding certain foods, alcohol and dangerous drugs; or taking prescribed medication to lower blood pressure or cholesterol. Taking proper care of oneself has become a modern virtue to rival the importance of taking care of others.

Those who sell things or otherwise try to manipulate human behavior learned long ago that people respond to certain stimuli at some primal level. Sampling any evening's television fare reveals that images of sexually attractive women are one stimulus that is employed repeatedly. Another series of messages exploit concern about health, especially to promote foods, drugs or other products claiming to enhance it. The scholarly study of decision making under conditions of uncertainty has revealed the remarkable extent to which individuals tend to make irrational choices in situations that are described in terms of human lives possibly being lost. A push on the longevity button triggers a response at some deeper level of our basic humanity. Unfortunately, this fact is well known.

This means that people are bombarded with a constant stream of longevity and health messages. Some are well-meaning efforts by health authorities to modify lifestyles. Others are intended to increase the profits of companies that sell food, drugs or other products. With disturbing frequency it is impossible to tell these apart: public service advertisements about the importance of taking blood pressure medicine were secretly funded by a company that sold these drugs. Cholesterol lowering was promoted by a food company to increase its sales. This means that the daily torrent of health and longevity information is contaminated by conflicts of interest and, more often than not, is fragmentary and misleading. The main problem is not accuracy but motive. Information intended to alter behavior is, almost by definition, oversimplified and lacking in balance. It is propaganda or advertising. Without a larger perspective on longevity and some basic tools to judge which hazards need to be dealt with and which may be ignored, it is difficult to make wise decisions about the risks of everyday life. The extreme but simple solutions are not appealing. To worry about every conceivable risk means spending a lifetime afflicted with unnecessary anxiety about health. To proceed with reckless abandon may needlessly squander life to no useful purpose or possible gain.

The study of life expectancy, however, is not merely an exercise with practical value. The subject is inherently fascinating. To think about the human lifespan is to wonder who we are and what we might become; to guard against dangers that imperil us and rejoice at those we have tamed; to probe for the secrets of success in prolonging life and measure the potential costs of failure. It is a story that stretches from the dawn of human history into the mists of possible futures. The first installment of this story consists of a reconnaissance of the entire territory, a sweeping look at the most important concepts, issues and questions that will be explored throughout this book.

Even during the four most recent decades, the continuous improvement in life expectancy is impressive. In the United States since 1950, the chances of dying in the next year have been reduced by more than 35 percent. Furthermore, these gains have been spread all across the age spectrum. Among newborns, the risk of dying in the first year has been reduced 81 percent. The mortality rate for stroke, an important cause of death among the elderly, has declined 61 percent. Accidents are the major peril to those neither old nor very young. The accidental death rate—everything from automobile and aircraft accidents to falls, drowning and fires—has been reduced by 39 percent. The notable exception to this broad trend is the slow but steady increase in cancer mortality. Expressed in terms of life expectancy, the overall gain was more than five years. But in contrast to previous periods, much of the improvement came among those over 50 years old, rather than among infants and children.

So constant is the exploitation of public fears about potential health hazards that it is easy to overlook the more basic fact that modern life has become remarkably safe. In the United States today, for example, 99 percent of those who reach their first birthday will also celebrate their twenty-fifth birthday. It will be difficult to improve greatly upon the remarkable record achieved among 10-year-old boys and girls. Of every 10,000 such children alive today, 9,998 will reach age 11. Probably no other living creatures in history have achieved survival rates found among young children in advanced democracies. Also, it speaks volumes to remember that a century and a half ago, more than 1 out of 3 children would be dead by age 10.

Such excellent prospects are not limited to young children benefiting from the constant vigilance of parents and a protective society. The outlook for the middle-aged—especially those with only modest longevity advantages—is also impressive. In the United States, a white 45-year-old woman in good health who doesn't smoke can expect to reach age 88, a comparable male, age 82.

The safety of modern-day life is illustrated in a story that physician and educator Richard W. Riegelman tells of his early professional days as a young doctor. He first practiced medicine with the health maintenance organization at George Washington University in Washington, D.C. The GWU health plan provided comprehensive medical care to university students and faculty, and was also popular among thousands of young professionals and their families. The physicians were organized into teams that cared for several thousand patients.

"I practiced medicine for ten years with only one death occurring among the patients in our entire group. I remember this vividly because we were quite shocked when a patient, a faculty colleague, died of cancer." Such are the realities of being a young adult in an era when life expectancy exceeds 75 years.

Unfortunately, life expectancy at birth is not an accurate measure of how long anyone in particular might reasonably expect to live. On its face, life expectancy at birth is treacherously simple. It reports the average age at death—and therefore typical lifespan—of everyone who died during a particular time period, usually one year. However, any specific figure likely understates the life expectancy of a majority to whom it is usually applied. The reason is somewhat subtle. Life expectancy is a composite snapshot of the mortality rates observed during one single year. But we live our lives over many years. Since over recent decades, those mortality rates have steadily declined, we can expect to live most of our life at lower death rates than those reported for this particular year.

Life expectancy at birth probably understates most people's chances for a second reason. Incorporated into the one-year snapshot are the risks of living through all ages, from birth onward. Having already survived the vulnerability of infancy, the hazards of adolescence, and other risks, adults have better prospects. This is an easier problem to solve than guessing the mortality rates over future decades. Separate life expectancy calculations are computed and published for every age. For example, if life expectancy at birth is 75 years, it will grow to 82 years among those who reach age 40. As you age, the number of years of life remaining is steadily reduced, but as a survivor you get farther and farther ahead of the population average, which includes all those who did not live as long as you already have.

However, this upbeat outlook for improved life expectancy depends on the key assumption that the slow but steady progress observed over many decades continues without major interruption. This 150-year-long growth curve is so central to modern human life expectancy that a major section of this book will examine the interplay of forces that produced these extraordinary gains. The most important factor is a seemingly familiar one—infectious disease. However, as later chapters will show, the role of microscopic life-forms remains of great significance in human affairs and exercises important influence over the prospects for life expectancy in the future.

By an accident of design, life expectancy figures conceal an underlying trend that is essential to any serious discussion of longevity. It is one of those central facts of life we all know but often overlook. Life expectancy was described earlier as a snapshot of all the mortality rates in effect in a particular year. Such a snapshot is needed because these rates vary so widely by age.

The first 12 months of life are about five times riskier than the years that immediately follow. In fact, mortality rates continue to drop steadily to reach, in modern times, a rock bottom minimum at age 10. Then a very slow rise begins, so gradual that, as noted earlier, only 1 percent of those who reach age 1 will have died by age 25. Moving along the exponential growth curve, death rates begin to increase relentlessly:

Age	Time until 1 percent die
1	25 years
25	7 years
42	2 years
50	1 year
70	4 months
80	2 months

This is a pattern worth pausing to absorb, a relationship so vital it is hard to think of a more central fact of life itself. Demographers and insurance actuaries call this awesome trend the force of mortality; the biological term is senescence. It means that with increasing age the organism becomes increasingly vulnerable to damage. With senescence an organism succumbs to the very same hazards that caused little harm at earlier ages. In the language of numbers, the exponential increase means that mortality rates double about every eight years. Early in adult life, the base mortality rates are so low that doubling them is barely perceptible. Late in life, the death rate is so high that no one survives past age 115.

The risks of life are sometimes quoted to the public as if this central trend either didn't exist or wasn't important enough to consider. For example, promoters of public safety might quite accurately advertise that auto accidents are the largest cause of death among teenagers aged 15–17. Watchful parents might be well advised to guard against the greatest single risk to their son's or daughter's life, which is in fact driving a car. But we also know intuitively that the absolute annual risk of accidental death is reasonably low, in this case about 1 in 3,000. This is one reason that teenagers drive despite the risks. For perspective, it is also important to remember that the danger of accidents looms so important among teenagers in part because other risks are extremely small. Measured over one year, these youths have an amazingly low risk of dying of the major causes of deaths: coronary heart disease (1 chance in 2 million), cancer (1 chance in 25,000) and infectious disease (1 chance in 1 million). Watching a teenager in action often does not always convey that same sense of invulnerability, but as a robust biological system, we've practically never seen anything like it.

This discussion has already illustrated that most lines of inquiry into the influences on life expectancy rapidly end up examining mortality rates directly. They are building blocks, when examined by age group, out of which the overall life expectancy figure is constructed. However, mortality rates don't have an intrinsic meaning that can be immediately grasped. For example, in 1987, the age-adjusted mortality rate in the United States was 535.5 per 100,000, or more simply 0.5 percent. This is the functional equivalent of a life expectancy of 74.8 years. Not only do rates have so little intrinsic meaning, they also vary so widely by age.

Therefore many scientific studies—and also this book—often leave out the actual numbers and simply cite differences for comparison. (For example, it was reported earlier that since 1950 the overall mortality rate had declined by more than 35 percent without mentioning the actual figures.) It is usually simpler to examine mortality rates by comparison— as long as one remembers how dramatically these rates vary by age. A 50 percent drop in coronary heart disease mortality rates among teenagers is an event of limited significance, a difference of about 150 deaths nationwide; among 60-year-olds, where the risks are nearly 2,000 times greater, such a reduction would be a major development. The search for important influences on life expectancy, therefore, focuses primarily on differences in mortality rates.

Among those living in the advanced democracies today, striking contrasts in longevity may be observed. Few factors are inherently so simple and offer so few ambiguities as cigarette smoking. It represents a clear benchmark against which other influences may be measured. One of the largest and longest studies of smoking involved determining the smoking status of one million middle-class men and women, and then following them for the next 12 years. It was sponsored by the American Cancer Society and directed by Edward A. Lew, a public-spirited insurance actuary who has written extensively about life expectancy. Among men, for example, it showed that the mortality rate among those who smoked a pack a day was more than twice as high as among those who had never smoked. Among those 35–45 years old, it reduced life expectancy by seven years; by age 70 the difference had declined to slightly less than three years. A smaller study based on a national sample of 1986 death certificates reached equally sobering conclusions. Among women who reached age 25, for example, 45 percent of heavy smokers died before age 70, compared with only 15 percent of nonsmokers. It is possible that other habits or characteristics common to smokers, besides the direct effect of tobacco, may account for some of the excess mortality that is observed. But there is little doubt the effect is real and important. It has even been observed in smoking studies of identical twins.

Few influences on life expectancy reach this magnitude. Further, it is even rarer to observe such analytical simplicity, a precisely defined pattern of behavior of which individuals may choose to partake. Most other lifestyle questions are plagued by measurement problems, questions of cause and effect, and other difficulties. Longevity is a subject graced by so few easy answers that it is helpful to begin with the essence of simplicity: A regular smoking habit doubles mortality rates.

Another important factor seems equally simple at first glance but doesn't turn out that way. Throughout Europe, the United States and the Pacific rim, women outlive men by large margins. In Greece women live five years longer than men, in Japan six years, and in the United States seven years. In the former Communist bloc countries the differences loom larger still: eight years in Hungary, and a staggering ten-year gap in the republics of the former Soviet Union. The pattern is so universal that in only one country in the world, Nepal, do men live longer than women, and there they have a one-year advantage.

These differences exist even though in any given community men and women share roughly the same housing, food, medical system, sanitary conditions and immunization practices. One might suppose that perhaps men engage in life-shortening behaviors that women forgo. However, there are truly enormous variations in sex roles, diet, lifestyle and behavior among the nations, while this difference is universally observed. In Japan hardly any women smoke, and a large majority of men do. In the United States the smoking habit is less prevalent among men and more evenly divided between the sexes. Large sex differentials in longevity are found in countries where most married women are in the work force, for example, the former Soviet Union and the United States. They are also found in those where a majority are not, for example, Italy and Japan.

This leads one to suspect that here it is mainly a case of biological differences. They are obvious to the eye and increase under additional scrutiny. Some disorders such as muscular dystrophy affect only men, and can be tracked precisely to that missing segment of DNA, left out in the Y chromosome of men, but included in duplicate copies on the two Xs of women. Hormonal differences may explain women's low susceptibility to coronary heart disease until menopause and provide other advantages. This kind of analysis tends to lead firmly toward the biological camp, suggesting a matter of genetics and heredity rather than environment, a gift of nature rather than a primary result of nurture. If those biological secrets could be unraveled, an additional seven years of life for men would be an extraordinary gain.

One fact transforms this entire discussion. Throughout most of human history, women have had the same or a shorter lifespan. This was true in the Bronze Age, in ancient Greece and republican Rome, in medieval Hungary, and in Italy as recently as 1891. The steady growth in the female advantage began roughly 150 years ago and appears to be continuing. Declines in deaths associated with childbirth contributed but by no means explain the differences. They are also observed with many other causes, including infectious disease, cancer and heart disease. Biological differences between males and females did not change over the past century. The transformation occurred in how human society was organized, and in its relationship with nature.

The reasons women live much longer than men, therefore, must involve the interaction of all these forces, of which the most important must be quite basic elements of human society observed over many differing cultures. It may be that during centuries of evolution women evolved as tougher, more resilient organisms capable of withstanding the trauma of childbirth and the additional stresses of primary care for children. When modern society reduced some of those burdens, the advantages remained. The problem with that explanation, however, is that a century and a half ago women were also more vulnerable than men to tuberculosis, pneumonia and other infectious disease, and these once important diseases struck hardest in childhood and early adulthood before marriage and childbearing years began. Women didn't appear more resilient, as they do today; they seemed weaker, sicker and more vulnerable. The mortality data provide at least some factual support for the social prejudices of the time. This suggests that as human society produces increasingly healthy and more resilient people who survive longer, it has somehow been more successful with women than men. For now, however, the difference remains a puzzle that nevertheless illustrates dramatically that lifespan is always an interaction between the innate biological characteristics of an organism and the environment in which it is nurtured.

To find another well-defined group with unusually good prospects for a long life, one need search no further than the United States Army or Air Force. Not only are mortality rates spectacularly low in the military services, but also the contrast with the general population raises an entirely new set of questions about life expectancy. Here seems to be a difference in lifespan even larger than that observed for the two other major factors, smoking and sex. Measured in the peacetime years of 1981–83, Army servicemen had a mortality rate that was 43 percent lower than the general population; in the Air Force the rate was 54 percent lower. Not only was this contrast found among robust young recruits, it was sustained with advancing age. While the military mortality data don't prove the old aphorism that old soldiers never die, it seems to come close. The mortality rate of military officers of age 50 or older was 76 percent lower than the general population of the same age. That is one of the most dramatic differences to be found in any mortality data.

Does this mean that enlisting in the military is the way to achieve a long and healthy life? In fact, it demonstrates something else entirely. Only healthy individuals are accepted into military service. Those who develop health problems during a military career, or even because of it, are discharged. It is the classic example of selection bias. This is called the *healthy worker effect* and it can be observed among practically any group of employed men and women. Consider, for example, a 1991 study trying to identify possible long-term effects of radiation on workers at the nuclear weapons facility at Oak Ridge, Tennessee. Teasing out any ill effects was difficult because the workers monitored for radiation had a mortality rate that was only 63 percent that of the general population of the same age. One would not, presumably, conclude that working with radioactive materials improved life expectancy. What the study demonstrates is that any group of healthy, able-bodied workers will have a substantially longer life expectancy than the general population. This occurs because a small but unfortunate minority is included among the general adult population, but is mostly excluded from the ranks of the full-time employed. The minority are those with seriously impaired health. Every age group includes those with life-shortening disorders, including muscular dystrophy, multiple sclerosis, heart disease and cancer. Since a large share of the premature deaths will occur among those with already impaired health, this reduces the average life expectancy of the general population (where they are included) but not the group of full-time workers (where most with impaired health are excluded).

The selection bias of the healthy worker effect creates few misunderstandings because people rarely choose employment for its effect on longevity. However, many of the same problems are embedded in the evidence supporting fervently promoted benefits of exercise. Consider the problems raised by an important study frequently cited as the most authoritative evidence for the health recommendations. It was conducted among 17,000 Harvard alumni who were followed for 12 to 16 years. Lifetime exercise habits were determined by a single questionnaire that inquired about the time spent at leisure-time sports, the number of stairs climbed daily and the total distance walked.

The study compared Harvard graduates of all ages who exercised regularly and vigorously with those who were the least active. The vigorous exercisers were defined as those whose weekly exercise included 20 miles of walking, 7 hours of light sports, or the equivalent of some combination of walking, climbing stairs and sports. Then the mortality rates were compared. The vigorous exercisers' mortality rate was 28 percent lower than for those least active.

Assuming for the moment that the study is technically without important flaws, the larger and more interesting task is exploring what this finding means. Do we conclude, as did the authors of the study, that this demonstrates the health benefits of exercise? Or are those inherently healthy and robust more likely to be vigorously active—the exercise equivalent of the healthy worker effect? Even worse, are the differences partly an artifact created because the health-impaired minority with cancer, stroke, diabetes, arthritis and most other serious disabilities were included among the more sedentary? (The authors excluded only those diagnosed with coronary heart disease.) The suspicion of selection bias is strengthened when one observes that the difference was most dramatic among the oldest Harvard graduates, those over age 60. Among these men the mortality rate was 49 percent lower. Those performing the exercise equivalent of 7 hours of sports a week in their 60s and 70s and 80s cannot represent the typical health status of that population group. This didn't stop the authors from leaping to the opposite conclusion— that the benefits of exercise appear to increase with age.

These points need not diminish any satisfaction that vigorous exercisers may take in their superior health status and enhanced longevity prospects. They still fall into a group likely to live longer. But those considering devoting more of their time to exercise should not mistake this for evidence that their life expectancy will benefit from doing so. At older ages exercise may help arrest atrophy of the muscles, but its effect on longevity remains undetermined. On this evidence, therefore, we cannot say whether exercise is a cause of good health, or an effect of it, nor how much of the observed difference is explained, not by the benefits of physical activity, but by the simple exclusion of the overtly unhealthy.

If this is the evidence, how then did exercise become one of the major modern commandments for virtuous healthy living? A major section of this book will explore how control of weight, blood pressure and cholesterol became the centerpiece of the modern-day medical strategy for prolonging life. To see why factors of inherently modest significance were made to seem so important involves not only examining these risk factors themselves, but the people and organizations that have promoted them.

Meanwhile, just three factors—good health, smoking status, and the female sex—take us a long way toward answering the question, Who are the longest-lived people today? The search need not extend to the remote villages of the Caucasus or the residents of some hidden Shangri-La. Most of the longest-lived people the world has ever known are right around us. They are nonsmoking men who are employed and women in good health who don't smoke. Both have average lifespans in the 80s; many will live much, much longer. Throughout the book numerous other factors will be considered—genetic inheritance, obesity, diet, blood pressure, cholesterol level, education, occupation and marital status. Few will approach the explanatory power of these basics.

Even larger differences in average lifespan may be observed among entire nations. Life expectancy today ranges from an all-time, worldwide high of 79 years in Japan, to a low of 39 years in the central African nation of Chad. However short its life expectancy may seem, Chad still has more than double the average length of life found throughout most of the last 100,000 years of human existence. The longest lifespans in world history are found throughout the advanced democracies of western Europe, North America and Asia. Switzerland, at 78 years, places a close second to Japan. Virtually all the rest of the advanced, industrialized world falls into a narrow life expectancy zone of 75 to 77 years. The United States falls at the bottom of the zone, with 28 nations having a longer life expectancy. (That comparison, however, counts tiny entities such as Liechtenstein, Bermuda and Macao.) While there are several dozen members, this is nevertheless a very select club. Achieving a 75-year average lifespan constitutes an important social and cultural achievement never observed before present times, and found in only a small fraction of modern-day nations.

So how is this difficult feat accomplished? So striking is the diversity in race, social custom, diet, income and culture among the longest-lived nations, the main challenge is to find any characteristics these success stories share in common. What do Japan, Cyprus, Austria and the tiny Caribbean island of Montserrat share except a life expectancy of 77 years or more? In terms of racial heritage, the longevity leaders include Asians, northern Europeans, a Mediterranean people, and in Montserrat a population primarily of African origin. In size and geography, the leaders range from a tiny tropical Caribbean dependency with 12,000 inhabitants to a northern hemisphere Asian giant with 125 million population.

The longest-lived nations eat enormously different diets—although all offer plenty of calories. The leader of the pack, Japan, has a diet very low in saturated fat and other animal products and low in fat of any kind. The second longest-lived nation, Switzerland, has more animal fat in its diet than virtually any country in the world, except Austria, another long-lived nation. Sharing third place is Greece, with a diet based on olive oil or monosaturated fat. This suggests the longest lifespans the world has ever known are compatible with all three major dietary patterns, providing that nutrition is complete, abundant and widely available.

Included in the first ranks of longevity are tightly structured societies such as Japan and Spain and the less constrained social orders of the United States, Denmark and Sweden. Births to unmarried women are one simple measure of the social character of a country. In tradition-oriented Japan just 1 percent of all children are born out of wedlock, while in wide-open Sweden 50 percent of births are to unmarried women.

The longest-lived nations have medical systems that vary greatly in cost. The United States, while near the bottom of the advanced nation group in life expectancy, boasts the most expensive medical system in the world—by a large margin. Measured per person, the German system costs only half as much as the United States', the Japanese only 45 percent, and Greece's only one-tenth as much. All have the same or better life expectancy. However, virtually all the medical systems provide ready access to physicians with basically similar training. The differences begin after that point.

What the long-lived nations share may come as something of a surprise. Every single one except Cuba is a democracy. Communist functionaries, tin-pot dictators and military juntas cannot build societies providing the health and longevity of free democratic nations, a rule broken just once. And every one has a robust free-enterprise economic system, although government expenditures typically amount to from one-quarter to one-half of total economic output. The common thread of democracy recalls Francis Fukayama's striking observation that there has apparently never been a war between two liberal democracies. Even before the final collapse of the Communist world, an international health survey had concluded that life expectancy in those nations had been slowly declining for decades. The collapse was a self-evident economic failure, but the deterioration of health status and longevity began many years before.

In all long-lived nations except Israel, women bear fewer than two children on the average. Among the major long-lived nations, the lowest fertility rate occurs in former West Germany, with 1.4 births per woman of reproductive age; in most of the advanced countries the fertility rate is around 1.7 births. Israel stands alone as a notable exception, with a 77-year life expectancy but a fertility rate of 2.95. In a nearly universal pattern that may be observed across time and geography, the number of children per family declines after life expectancy rises and infant mortality falls.

Next to democracy and fertility, prosperity is the best predictor of a high life expectancy, but it is by no means an infallible guide. All the 10 richest nations of the world have achieved life expectancies of over 75 years. And none of the 10 poorest rises above 50 years. But beyond the extremes, notable discrepancies may be found: Hong Kong, Spain and Greece, for example, have achieved a better life expectancy with only one-third the per capita income of the United States. The economies of the former Communist countries of Hungary and Czechoslovakia out-performed the democracies of Spain and Greece, but their life expectancy trailed far behind.

Thus, people live longest in peaceful, relatively prosperous free democracies, mostly in the northern hemisphere. They live lengthy lives packed densely together in the metropolitan confines of Hong Kong, and scattered thinly across the vast expanses of Canada and Australia. Long-lived nations can be found on tropical Caribbean islands and in arctic cold of Iceland and Finland.

The causes of death also vary greatly among nations with a similar life expectancy. Consider the two leaders, Japan and Switzerland. The death rate for the leading killer in Switzerland—coronary heart disease—is three times higher than in Japan. But the Swiss suffer strokes at only half the rate the Japanese do and die of stomach cancer at only one-fifth the Japanese rate. Large disease-specific differences, especially in coronary heart disease, can be found throughout the longer-lived nations of the world. But the overall life expectancy is similar. They share in common the pattern that most deaths are caused by chronic diseases and accidents rather than by infectious disease. Heart disease is steadily declining throughout almost all these nations, and cancer is slowly increasing.

Different cultures, diets, medical systems, gene pools and disease patterns appear to produce remarkably similar mortality rates. A useful perspective is to consider longevity a complex end result—a sum that is greater than any of its individual parts. The great achievement of these long-lived nations has been a stable, prosperous environment in which healthy, robust people are nurtured. They are generally protected, particularly during infancy and childhood, from disease, violence, neglect, abuse and malnutrition. They grow taller, run faster, leap higher and live longer than any humans before.

None of these factors, however, provides even a hint at possible answers to a more profound question. Why are humans limited to a maximum lifespan of approximately 115 years? With literally billions of people alive under widely different conditions, why do not even a fortunate one or two survive until age 150 or 200? What explains the irreversible upward sweep of the increasingly lethal force of mortality?

We share the same fundamental biological design and long stretches of DNA with other mammals of widely varying lifespans: mice are claimed by the same force of mortality at just 27 months; dogs rarely live beyond 20 years; horses rarely survive past their 30s. What brings down the curtain of life at these particular intervals?

To examine possible answers to the question, consider an extended analogy that captures the fundamental issues. Suppose we were designing a spacecraft intended to reach the planet Mars and photograph it as it passes by. Such a spacecraft might have some components likely to wear out during the several years' journey to Mars. That limitation could be solved by providing replacements for the most vulnerable parts, or conceivably an on-board factory to manufacture the most perishable items. In the human counterpart, the stem cells of the bone marrow manufacture a steady new supply of red and white blood cells. The spacecraft would also require one or two power sources and communications and might carry other experiments on board.

Such a vehicle would require a control program, just as humans operate under programmed instructions encoded in DNA. Perhaps just before reaching Mars it would need instructions to deploy its precious camera and a special antenna. Humans, of course, undergo an even more radical programmed transformation upon reaching sexual maturity. The control program might also set priorities, especially if trouble occurred. For example, in a power shortage, it might shut down the most expendable equipment, just as human circulatory systems will deprive peripheral parts of the body of blood to protect the heart, lungs, kidneys and brain. At the center of our analogy is a control program that has a clear mission and that manages components with varying life expectancies of their own.

Now comes the most interesting question. Once the spacecraft has reached Mars and photographed it, concluding its mission, what happens next? In evolutionary terms, a similarly programmed mission is accomplished when we have reproduced and raised our young. That task requires a lifespan of 30 or 40 years, a fraction of what is typically achieved today. It might be that over hundreds of thousands of years evolution might favor societies with lifespans longer than the biological minimum because the older population provided better continuity, knowledge and leadership. It might also be that evolution favors the most robust and active societies that were the least burdened by the older, slower and less physically able. However, it seems most likely that after achieving the biological mission set by nature and evolution and programmed into our genes, we are simply on our own. The desire to cherish, preserve and prolong each individual life indefinitely seems a uniquely human objective.

What, then, happens to the spacecraft when it has photographed Mars, or to humans when they have reproduced and raised their young? The simplest explanation of the biological bonus of longevity is an idea called overinsurance. A spacecraft built to be certain to survive the enormous demands of a lengthy voyage to Mars is so well constructed that it is likely to operate indefinitely after accomplishing its mission. In fact, one of the Voyager spacecraft is operating 18 years after completing its mission of visiting the red planet. It is easy to imagine a similar kind of overinsurance in the design of a species requiring 13 to 15 years of nurturing and protection before reaching reproductive age.

To probe more deeply into the analogy, consider how the control program of the spacecraft might be designed. With mission accomplished, it is quite possible that the device would "run out of program." It would issue no more preserving and coordinating instructions, having no mission to preserve and no goal for which to safeguard resources. Presumably such a spacecraft would continue to operate until the first critical component failed, whether or not there were backup systems. There would be no particular point to devising a series of control instructions when the spacecraft no longer serves a purpose. In the landmark work *The Biology of Senescence,* author Alex Comfort uses the example of the World War II buzz bombs the Germans launched at England in the closing days of the war. One might wonder what the buzz bomb guidance program might do when it had passed its target, but failed to strike it, notes Comfort. Whatever happens is of no importance. The device had run out of program; the weapon's designer simply didn't care what happened if it didn't strike the target.

A more ominous-sounding possibility might in fact be the most promising in terms of extending the human lifespan. What if the spacecraft were programmed to destroy itself upon completing or failing its mission—as rockets and spacecraft are sometimes designed. The finality with which the curtain falls on humans at 115 years hints at a biological clock whose time has run out. The human body includes an intricate system of timing devices that control our transformation from fetus to adult; they regulate sleep and other cycles. The idea that programmed self-destruction is embedded in mankind's future may at first appear unpleasant and fatalistic. But a closer look reveals that the idea has almost magical allure. To suppose that a biological clock times human existence opens the door immediately to the idea of resetting that clock. Biologists have already identified and can alter the hormonal signals that halt growth and begin sexual maturity. Is it possible to identify—and therefore neutralize—the signals that call for our destruction? Later in this book, these kinds of questions will be explored in depth in the section on the science of longevity. It examines, among other things, biological clocks, free radicals, hormones with antiaging properties and techniques that extend the lifespan of mammals.

The force of mortality shapes the phases of our later life as surely as development and sexual maturity define our early years, interlocking pieces of the human life plan. The issues involved are so central and fascinating that they are surpassed perhaps only by the greatest of all mysteries of life: How the world's remarkable cornucopia of living creatures came to exist in the first place. As the next chapter will show, some of the smallest and simplest creatures ever to live on earth still play a crucial role in the longevity of humans.

CHAPTER TWO

A BATTLE JOINED

It is 9 A.M. at Washington Hospital Center in the nation's capital. In a tiny second floor room furnished with plain steel desks, Nancy Donegan, registered nurse, is getting ready to join the oldest of all ongoing human conflicts, the battle with microscopic forms of life. In the search for the important influences on human longevity, Nancy Donegan's hospital activities on this day will provide unexpected and revealing insights.

Washington Hospital Center lies 27 blocks due north of the gleaming white dome of the United States Capitol. A six-story jumble of towers, additions and discontinuous corridors, it mirrors in bricks and glass the rapid but haphazard growth of modern medical technology. In this medical citadel, modern mankind has assembled its most potent defenses against an invading army of bacteria, parasites, fungi and viruses. It will be Nancy Donegan's task this day to patrol the perimeters, hunting for microscopic life-forms seeking a permanent foothold, an opportunity to spread among the patients occupying the 907 beds of Washington Hospital Center.

Donegan's official title is managing director of the infection control department. Through the door of the hospital every day come numerous individuals harboring organisms whose survival depends upon their capacity to spread to others. Helping prevent this spread is one of Donegan's jobs. In addition, medical procedures performed at the hospital open new avenues to infection by breaching the body's natural defenses with an awesome variety of needles, catheters and other invasive devices. Therefore special protection is required. Donegan's third

major task is less obvious. Some microorganisms love hospitals, and
multiply and prosper despite an environment deliberately designed to be
inhospitable to them. These hospital-based bugs are either rarely found
or seldom dangerous elsewhere and are Donegan's sworn enemies.

Although medical authorities prefer not to advertise this fact, a modern hospital ranks high on the list of ideal targets for microscopic life-
forms. They flourish where a changing group of unrelated people spend
their days packed closely together. A complex with nearly a thousand
patients and more than four thousand employees easily meets this definition. An Army basic-training barracks and a school classroom are also
unusually hospitable to the rapid spread of microscopic predators. A
hospital also shelters a population of human beings so young their
immune systems have not yet fully developed, or so old their systems
have begun to decline, or so weak that body defenses have fallen below
the accustomed levels. Thus Washington Hospital Center is a place
where not only does Nancy Donegan go hunting for bugs, but bugs go
hunting for people. It is a mark of the power and adaptability of microscopic life-forms that they grow and prosper amidst mankind's most
active defenses. It is a hint of their power over the length of human life.

In a hospital world characterized by strictly defined hierarchal roles,
Nancy Donegan is one of the relatively few who have risen through the
ranks. A slender, compact woman with straight brunette hair and light
brown eyes, she abandoned a college English major for a nursing career
on grounds of practicality. Over the intervening years she rose from staff
nurse to head nurse, from head nurse to infection control practitioner,
from there to lead the day-to-day effort at infection control. She has a
daughter nine years old.

The first document to command Nancy Donegan's attention this
morning is called the isolation list. It is a one-page computer printout
listing the current patients with diseases that might readily spread to
others. In a city such as Washington, in this day and age, the list includes
many patients with AIDS. While it stands at the top of the list in terms
of mortal threats, AIDS is fairly difficult to transmit. Nevertheless, AIDS
patients do not share rooms except with other AIDS patients. Gloves are
worn routinely for personal contact, with precautions escalating to
gowns and glasses for surgery or other kinds of invasive procedures
where blood or other body fluids might splash. The hospital environ-

ment is loaded with needles, syringes, scalpels and catheters—equipment that staff call "sharps." A needle stick puncture while helping an AIDS patient carries a 1 in 300 chance of transmitting the disease. A plain orange card beside the hospital room door of each AIDS patient advises the initiated to exercise precautions against infectious diseases that are transmitted by blood or body fluids.

While Donegan expresses no special concern at the many AIDS patients on the isolation list, even a single case of another disease would instantly trigger the loudest of alarms. An infection control headache of epic proportions would immediately begin if the hospital had admitted a patient—or worse yet discovered an employee—with one of the most familiar of all human diseases, the measles virus. The nightmare of measles is the extraordinary ease with which it can be transmitted. Exposure is defined as anyone who occupied the same air space—for example, an elevator or hospital room—within two hours of the time a person with measles was present. To make matters even more difficult, someone infected with measles is highly contagious for at least four days before the characteristic rash first appears.

"I have to find out not only who Suzi saw on Saturday, Sunday, Monday, and Tuesday," Donegan says, "but who came in after she was in the area."

Since the introduction of a vaccine in 1963, the incidence of measles has been reduced from half a million cases each year to a few thousand. It remains, however, a hospital hazard because in the early years of vaccination there were numerous cases where the vaccine proved ineffective, and many individuals remain unaware of their vulnerability. The hospital is also populated with infants too young to be vaccinated, and those whose immune systems have been compromised by advanced age, by AIDS, by organ transplants or by cancer treatment.

Fortunately, on this day there are no measles cases on Nancy Donegan's isolation list. However, the contrast between the two diseases, measles and AIDS, provokes an important question about a virus that has not yet appeared on the isolation list of any hospital, anywhere in the world. What would happen if nature produced a virus that combined the deadly characteristics of AIDS, and its capacity to disarm the immune system, with measles' extraordinary facility to leap from person to person, riding on the tiniest, microscopic particles of dust or moisture?

It can be said with some confidence that such a disease would inevitably kill a large fraction of the human race, and might extinguish the species altogether. The possibility of such a disease ranks far up the scale of plausibility from the speculations of science fiction and fantasy writers. As subsequent chapters will show, the immutable force of evolution pushes neither viruses nor humans toward that particular biological Armageddon. But sooner or later nature tries everything. This is why the possibility that the AIDS virus in particular might mutate into a more transmissible form already has produced an exchange now legendary in the annals of scientific repartee.

Joshua Lederberg, the Nobel laureate in physiology and medicine, was the keynote speaker at a Washington, D.C., conference on emerging viruses in May 1989. Lederberg is one of the bright lights of the world of biology, and was about to conclude a lengthy term as president of Rockefeller University. During the session he raised the possibility that a mutation of the AIDS virus might permit its transmission by aerosol droplets.

He was immediately challenged by a world-renowned expert on the molecular structure of that virus, Howard Temin of the University of Wisconsin, who is also a Nobel Prize winner.

"I think we can very confidently say this can't happen," said Temin. However, he did concede that the AIDS virus could change its structure enough to be transmitted through the air. "Then we might have a virus that could be spread by the respiratory route, but it would no longer cause AIDS. It might be just another cold virus."

Lederberg retorted, "I don't share your confidence about what can and cannot happen."

Temin persisted in an argument that became increasingly technical. Theoretically anything is possible, he said, "But you don't have to stay up nights worrying about it."

Lederberg said, "I'm glad that I worry enough for both of us, Howard."

Throughout history, the life expectancy of human beings has been regulated by a relationship with life-forms of microscopic size. On occasion both war and famine have shortened human lives by the thousands and, more rarely, by the millions. However, a study of that fraction of human history for which systematic health records exist, and clues from the more dimly perceived past, reveals that microscopic predators dwarf all other factors as a cause of early and unexpected death. No war ever destroyed one-half of the population of entire continents or reduced the population of island communities by 90 to 100 percent. Disease has done so repeatedly. At least one famine, the potato famine of 1845–49, had a devastating impact in Ireland. But it was caused by a disease that attacked the food supply rather than people. One of the most destructive wars in history, World War I, claimed more than 7 million lives on the battlefield over four and a half years. The flu epidemic that swept the world in its wake killed 20 million much more quickly. Unfortunately, the three towering threats to human life expectancy—war, famine and disease—cannot be segregated in tidy and separate compartments. They are inextricably interrelated. Until recent times, approximately half the soldiers who died in war were felled by disease rather than the enemy. An early effect of malnutrition is increased susceptibility to disease. Usually the toll of war is not limited to the opposing armies; it often destroys crops and the transportation system that distributes food.

The long-term threats to human longevity should not be measured only by the spectacular but relatively rare apocalyptic events, whether plague, war or famine. As this and subsequent chapters will show, careful examination of the planet we share with trillions of microscopic life-forms reveals a relationship that is present everywhere, operating at all times, and always changing.

The overwhelming importance of microscopic life-forms in determining human life expectancy can be illustrated through several comparisons. In Britain and the United States, about 12 years were added to human life expectancy when the deadly lung diseases tuberculosis and pneumonia slowly receded. The complete elimination of the greatest health terror of the present, cancer, would add only two years to the average lifespan. In the United States during this century, neither war nor famine has ever reversed the steady improvement in life expectancy. But disease has done so repeatedly, the most recent example occurring in 1988. Deaths from three sources of disease are on the increase. Mortality is increasing rapidly from both AIDS and septicemia—the medical term for uncontrolled growth of microorganisms in the blood. And the century-long decline in pneumonia reversed in 1986. The overall pattern of disease mortality is one of slow, ceaseless ebb and flow, interrupted by periodic eruptions that ravage human life on a scale equaled by no other force of man or nature.

The most striking characteristic of the relationship between human beings and microscopic life-forms is the certainty of change. As one disease moderates, another may arise. A harmless bacterium, proliferating in practically any available pool of water, may turn into a killer under certain circumstances. A devastating plague may suddenly and mysteriously vanish, or slowly decline year by year.

Not only do diseases change constantly, so does the human environment in which they must live. To survive, a microscopic predator requires a continuous supply of vulnerable human or other hosts. Combine the extraordinary adaptability of microscopic life-forms with the modern human propensity for rapid change, and you have the mighty engine that sometimes extends and sometimes shortens human life expectancy. This chapter and the four chapters that follow will seek to portray the most important aspects of the titanic collision between those two forces.

The steady give and take of that relationship stands out in bold relief in the daily operations of every major hospital in the country. In a laboratory at Washington Hospital Center one important dimension of that relationship is illustrated.

Carol Ormes, the microbiology supervisor, is one of the few individuals at Washington Hospital Center who spend time trying to figure out how to keep bacteria healthy rather than killing them off. Unless they can be first made to grow in culture, bacteria cannot be identified. And that is her responsibility. In the bustling room next door to her office many of the 25 persons employed in the laboratory are at work on this process.

Bacteria are among the oldest, most ubiquitous and most successful life-forms on earth. They thrive on the hot sulfur that bubbles through volcanic vents in the deepest trenches of the ocean and can be found buried in the Arctic ice. As hardened spores, they can be found soaring in the stratosphere at an altitude of 32 miles. In evolutionary terms, bacteria had a two-billion-year head start on all plants and animals during the Archean era when they dominated the earth. In this context, the development of the enormously more complex cells in plants and animals must be regarded as a recent innovation.

One group of bacteria have truly made the gift of life to all plants and animals on earth. The structural proteins in every animal and plant cell are constructed from the basic 20 amino acids, so named for the combination of two hydrogen atoms and one nitrogen atom that forms an essential component of all amino acids, and thus of all plants and animals. Although the atmosphere of the earth is four-fifths nitrogen, this bountiful source of supply is utterly useless to us in that form. All advanced life-forms require nitrogen-fixing bacteria to perform the pivotal task of combining one atom of nitrogen with two atoms of hydrogen required for amino acids. In humans, the bacteria's output is obtained through the protein in our diet.

There is hardly an imaginable niche in life that bacteria do not occupy. Both grazing animals and termites rely on bacteria to break down the cellulose in grasses into starch; no animal can perform this critical chemical task. Bacteria inhabit any handy pool of water, live by the billions in a spoonful of soil, and can be found proliferating on counter tops, doorknobs, mop buckets and window shades. It is not surprising that an astonishing variety of bacteria specialize in human beings. Unlike many other places on earth, the relationship is in no real sense mutually beneficial. At best they are harmless parasites in humans, at worst toxic and deadly predators.

In part because they are so simple—the basic molecular components of life floating free in a sea of cytoplasm—bacteria are capable of growing and changing with astonishing speed. A single *E. coli* bacterium, which inhabits the intestine, if provided the necessary nutrients, would multiply so quickly that in three days' time its descendants would weigh as much as the entire earth.

Bacteria, with their DNA floating freely in the cell's cytoplasm rather than confined in a specialized nucleus, have another advantage denied more complex life-forms. Segments of DNA can form tiny rings called plasmids. Not only do bacteria pass on these plasmids when the cell divides, but they also exchange plasmids with other bacteria through a process called conjugation. This capacity to evolve in literally a matter of days provides an enormous quantity of work for Carol Ormes and the other medical technicians at Washington Hospital Center.

Today Ormes will solve a straightforward identification problem. A hospital nurse has used a moistened cotton swab to collect microorganisms present in a skin infection in a patient in one of the intensive care units, and sealed it in a plastic tube. Using a wire loop, the bacteria had been transferred to a thin layer of nutrient medium spread across the surface of several petri dishes. Next the clear plastic plates had been incubated for 24 hours in a comfortably warm and moist environment. The microbiology laboratory is filled with stacks of these petri dishes, and Carol Ormes shuffles them with the same effortless, practiced skill with which a casino blackjack dealer handles a deck of cards.

She holds up a petri dish featuring a multicolored outbreak of bacterial growth resembling what one might find on a piece of cheese left in the refrigerator much too long.

"I can already tell you what that is," says Ormes, pointing to one large patch of luxuriant white growth, "but let's make sure." Ormes has spent 31 years in the microbiology laboratory and can spot some of the most serious repeat offenders on sight. But confirmation is still important.

She picks up a second plate, on which the same bacteria were being tested. The plate started out covered with a light red layer of a mixture called mannitol salt. The high salt content, about a 7 percent solution, will prevent a large majority of bacteria from growing—the reason salt is one of the oldest and simplest of preservatives. Most of the rest of the mixture is a form of sugar called mannitol. One particular species of bacteria feeds on this sugar, converting it to acid. If it should do so, a relative of the chemical in litmus paper changes color from light red to bright yellow. It is immediately obvious that more than half of this plate has turned bright yellow. Under a 100-power microscope countless round organisms are visible, looking like tiny clusters of grapes. Ormes has identified the always difficult and sometimes dangerous nemesis of all hospitals, *Staphylococcus aureus*.

It is one tough customer. It tolerates salt. Within limits, it doesn't mind heat. It can go without moisture for weeks and still remain alive. *Staph. aureus* can hitch rides on the surface of the skin, where it is harmless—and cling to clothing. But most often it lurks in the nose, hiding in the nasal passages, where it does little or no harm. About 80 percent of the population carries *Staph. aureus* at some time in their lives, and about 30 percent have harbored it continuously since birth.

Under many circumstances, it is an omnipresent, tough, persistent, but benign resident of the nasal passages. However, the exceptions are arresting. Perhaps the best-known example is toxic shock syndrome. A new brand of highly absorbent tampon provided the perfect environment for the normally present staph to multiply in large numbers. In itself, this could still be utterly harmless, but like other disease-causing bacteria, this variety of staph secretes several toxic substances—and different amounts under different conditions. In this case the staph secreted a toxin that caused a rapidly rising fever, skin rash, kidney failure and a sudden drop in blood pressure so severe that death sometimes resulted.

Staph. aureus and toxic shock syndrome provide an excellent illustration of a broader case in point. As the full scope of the relationship between human health, longevity and microscopic life-forms is explored in this and later chapters, one pattern will emerge repeatedly. Harmless organisms in one environment suddenly become deadly killers under another set of circumstances. This sequence of action and reaction explains both large gains and substantial losses in human life expectancy. The events that occurred the next day in Carol Ormes's laboratory will illustrate a second, equally important dimension to this relationship.

It is not enough simply to know the name of the enemy, especially one as tough and slippery as *Staph. aureus*. In fact, the next procedure is perhaps the most important step. Samples of the staph bacteria grown in the initial cultures are spread evenly in a nutrient medium across a larger clear plastic plate, this one 7 inches across. Then 12 circular disks, each about the size of a shirt button, are deposited at equal intervals, like candles spaced neatly on a birthday cake. This plate goes back into the incubator to nurture the bacteria.

Ormes holds up a plate to show what has happened over one day's time. One tiny button was impregnated with penicillin. On the surface of the plate the staph grow happily around it in the nutrient medium, utterly unaffected. This represents a kind of biological full circle because the dramatic effect of penicillin was first observed by Alexander Fleming in 1928 when he saw it had killed *Staph. aureus* growing on a petri dish much like this one. The really remarkable property, however, was that penicillin proved highly toxic to a wide array of bacteria but was utterly harmless to the cells of plants and animals. A critical difference in cellular structure explains how this occurs. A bacterial cell can be pictured as a bag of fluid protected by a rigid network of girders built out of carbohydrate molecules. Penicillin prevents bacteria, at cell division, from forming the chemical bonds needed to build this external skeleton. The cells of animals and plants have no such tough exterior skeleton, and are unaffected.

Only a few years after penicillin came into widespread use during World War II, the first reports appeared showing that a few strains of *Staph. aureus* had learned how to manufacture a protein called beta-lactamase that neutralized the toxic effects of penicillin.

Once the genetic blueprint for neutralizing penicillin existed, a simple experiment demonstrates what happened next. Grow a few million staph on a petri dish, and then add penicillin. First, the penicillin reduces the competition for food by killing most of the organisms without the resistance gene. Not only do the resistant bacteria multiply, they exchange their plasmid rings of DNA with other bacteria, so the resistant bacteria grow not only exponentially—but even faster. Today, the penicillin resistance first acquired in hospitals has spread throughout practically all the *Staph. aureus* bacteria in the world. Infectious disease specialists note with concern that *Staph. aureus* is demonstrating the capacity to exchange useful genetic instructions with a related but separate species, the even more plentiful *Staphylococcus epidermidis*.

The petri dish Carol Ormes holds in her hand has 12 buttons, representing 12 different antibiotic drugs. This particular staph can resist penicillin, erythromycin, tetracycline and seven other drugs, a total of 10. But surrounding just two of the buttons is a clear, 2-inch-wide ring of bacteria-free plastic where the drugs have killed off all the staph in their immediate neighborhood. While two antibiotics still kill this particular strain, the medical journals are filled with reports that sometimes staph can resist these two drugs as well.

Another troublesome hospital bacterial species, *Clostridium difficile*, can be described as the evolutionary child of broad-spectrum antibiotics. *C. difficile* can inhabit the intestinal tract of humans, seals, donkeys, hamsters and other animals. It is normally a minor player, mostly harmless among the hundreds of varieties of bacteria that flourish in the intestine, with its ideal combination of warmth, moisture and a steady supply of nutrients. While *C. difficile* acquired antibiotic resistance, this normally helped it little because of the heavy bacterial competition in the human gut. Antibiotic therapy changes that balance dramatically. With its competitors mostly killed off, *C. difficile* multiplies rapidly; in large numbers it secretes enough toxin to cause major intestinal problems.

While the bacteria identified in the microbiology laboratory can be extremely dangerous in patients, Ormes and the staff handle the petri dishes with much confidence and few special precautions. One notable exception will send them scurrying down the hallway to a room equipped with a special laboratory hood, negative air pressure and other safeguards: a specimen to be tested for tuberculosis. While tuberculosis is no longer a dreaded killer among the general public, TB bacteria retain their old characteristics of being among the toughest to kill and easiest to transmit of any the world has ever known. TB is also making a comeback, especially among AIDS victims, after acquiring resistance to the three major drugs used to combat it.

In another basement laboratory of Washington Hospital Center, John C. Rees, doctor of microbiology, is trying to identify a predator so tiny that a row of ten million could be lined up side-by-side on the head of a pin. It kills human cells. It has been found in mucus, blood, breast milk, urine, stool, tears and semen. To confirm or disprove his suspicions, Rees will employ the sophisticated tools of modern biotechnology. However, even if he finds the predator, it will not be possible to kill it. The quarry he stalks, a tiny viral particle, has never been alive. Even though constructed from the same organic molecules as living things, it lies clearly beyond the line that separates what is a living creature from what is not. Every living cell, from the most primitive bacterium to the most sophisticated optic sensor, conducts an endless and perfectly balanced series of chemical reactions, assembling and breaking apart molecules, acquiring and giving up energy in the process. Should these reactions cease, the cell dies. A virus does none of this.

It does, however, contain one or more molecules of nucleic acid with the genetic instructions, written in the common DNA code, for making another copy of itself. This entity, strictly speaking, is not entered into the great game of life; it contains only the directions for playing. The coded instructions are the only essential component of a virus. However, most have a protein coat that is sometimes studded with spikes. And some contain a molecule or two of some other key chemical. In large quantities some viruses look crystalline, and can be stored in a jar on the shelf for decades, like sugar.

Should it gain entry to a human cell, the virus diverts the complex machinery to a new purpose: making copies of itself. This works long enough to create hundreds to thousands of additional particles before it wrecks the host cell and is released to enter other cells. Some viruses, even the one Rees is hunting today, do not invariably destroy the host cell. These viruses may gain entry and lurk undetected for years doing no harm whatever. One great unsolved mystery is what suddenly makes latent viruses become active.

Rees, who heads the virology laboratory at Washington Hospital Center, has received a culture of sputum in a solution laced with antibiotics to kill off the bacteria. He can't grow this virus simply by feeding it nutrients. It requires the living cells of human beings.

From the freezer, Rees takes a plastic vial containing cancerous human lung cells. Cancer has disabled the controls that limit cell division to precisely defined conditions, and rapid reproduction occurs. However perilous inside the body, a culture of rapidly multiplying human cells is ideal for the virus. He introduces the possible viral particles to the human cells and waits to see how they get along during the next two days.

The viruses are much too tiny to see with an ordinary light microscope. But it is possible to observe whether a virus is beginning to destroy the host cells. Depending on the virus under study, the invaded cells may bulge, become oddly rounded or rupture as millions of virus particles come off the protein assembly line of the cell. Virologists call this cytopathic effect, or CPE.

Under a microscope, Rees examines a culture of some cancer cells introduced to a virus several days earlier. To the inexperienced eye, it looks like some of the cells are bigger and more rounded than their neighbors. It is obvious, however, that to identify a specific virus, or even be sure of the effect, requires experienced and disciplined powers of observation. In addition Rees will confirm this observation with an additional test.

He gets another small plastic vial filled with a clear liquid. Floating invisibly in the solution are millions upon millions of copies of one of the dazzling new products of biotechnology. They are called monoclonal antibodies. The antibodies, which Rees orders from the DuPont catalog, are a striking example of how far biotechnology has come. Antibodies, a critical component of the immune system, are Y-shaped molecules that circulate in the bloodstream of animals. When they encounter a distinctive molecular pattern that exactly mirrors its own, one of the top ends of the "Y" sticks to the virus or bacterium, much like an oddly shaped electrical plug that fits only into an exactly matching socket. The distinctive molecular pattern on a foreign substance is called an antigen. In the case of viruses, having antibodies attached may be sufficient to block the crucial maneuver of entering the cell. But the fit between antibody and the foreign antigen must be perfect. To this end millions of different antibodies circulate, each with the distinctive molecular pattern of some feature of a foreign substance.

The small vial contains millions of identical antibodies that match, specifically, a location on a specific viral particle he is stalking, and that virus alone. One additional modification has been made to these laboratory-bred, purified antibodies. A molecular side chain has been added to the shank of the "Y" of each antibody. Under fluorescent light it will glow bright green.

This time, the results are easy to see under a microscope. The antibodies have stuck hard to the viral particles, and the excess carefully washed away. Bright green areas may be seen clearly among the cells on the slide. Rees has confirmed the presence of cytomegalovirus, or CMV. At present, it is likely that a majority of the population has been successfully and permanently invaded by CMV.

In one study, 81 percent of the adult blood samples in Washington, D.C., tested positive for CMV; in another, 80 percent of the 55-year-olds in St. Petersburg. In Rochester, New York, only 38 percent of the adults were infected in 1966. But on the Caribbean Island of St. Lucia everyone tested has been infected. Unlike the more than 100 separate viruses that cause the common cold, this is not a virus that arrives, causes trouble, and is eliminated. CMV comes and stays forever, hiding inside cells where the antibodies patrolling in the bloodstream can't reach it.

Most of the time, most of the infected will never know they are sharing their cells with millions of viral particles. At birth, however, infection can result in hearing loss or other abnormal development in about 1 out of 3,000 cases. Those exposed to CMV for the first time in adolescence sometimes develop mononucleosis. Normally, the body cannot eliminate CMV infection, but it keeps it harmless. But destroy the delicate balance of the immune system, and CMV is an accident waiting to happen. It is especially difficult in AIDS cases and those who have received cancer chemotherapy.

Many viruses can gain entrance only to specific kinds of cells. Rabies, for example, infects only nerve cells. But CMV has been found in the retina, ears, lung, spleen, liver, heart and kidneys. Most often the effect is inflammation, sometimes accompanied by fever. Occasionally it is more severe; sometimes fatal.

Now that Rees has confirmed a viral infection there will be little else that can be done. The arsenal of weapons against the viral world is an extremely limited one. For some viruses there is a vaccine. For a small handful—for example, herpes and flu—there are drugs that can inhibit but not eliminate the infection. Acyclovir, for example, slows a CMV infection but the patient usually relapses as soon as treatment is halted. Overall, mankind's cupboard is surprisingly bare of tools to combat viruses. Hepatitis is a dangerous viral invasion of the liver; the ailing, however, are sent home because there is little that can be done for them in a hospital. Get an ordinary case of measles, and the staff will devoutly pray that the sufferer stays home. AIDS patients are treated aggressively in the hospital environment; but primarily to combat the bacterial and fungal invaders. Rees's virology lab at Washington Hospital Center can identify only three viruses: CMV and two kinds of herpes. The patient found infected with any of these three viruses cannot expect a cure. Samples where other viruses are suspected must be sent to even more elaborate and specialized laboratories. Combat with viruses is not primarily waged in a hospital, nor, as later chapters will show, is mankind a consistent victor.

An important dimension of the relationship between humans and microscopic life-forms is nearly invisible in the specialized environment of

Washington Hospital Center. Even without active human intervention, evolution does not inevitably promote development of increasingly lethal bacteria and viruses. A microscopic organism that instantly killed its host would quickly run out of hosts and would soon disappear. On the other extreme, some bacteria flourish through becoming harmless inhabitants of the skin, nose or intestine, becoming dangerous only when they are outside their normal habitat. Over long periods of time we can observe this process of constant adjustment between host and microscopic predator into a relationship tolerable to both. Those who study this mutual adjustment process often illustrate it with a remarkable case study involving rabbits.

As essential background for the rabbit story, we need to remember that for the last 100 million years, the Western Hemisphere and Australia were almost completely isolated from Europe and Asia. As a result, most animal life evolved on separate but sometimes parallel tracks. The now extinct liptotern of Argentina looked like a predecessor of the horse of Asia, but was in fact a completely separate evolutionary line. Australia developed neither horse species. The exact same pattern could be found among rabbits, with entirely separate species evolving in Europe and South America, but none in Australia.

Then in 1859 an overeager British colonizer introduced the rabbit into the ecological heaven of Australia. With an enormous food supply and no active competitors or predators, rabbits multiplied with astonishing speed, soon becoming a major pest. As early as 1888 Louis Pasteur proposed killing off the rabbits by deliberately introducing a disease, and in 1950 somebody actually tried it.

Rabbits in Brazil carry a harmless virus called myxomatosis, spread by mosquitoes. For many years nobody even noticed it—until European rabbits imported for use in experiments suddenly died of a mysterious disease. Once identified, myxomatosis turned out to have extraordinary lethality for European rabbits—nearly 99 percent—but was harmless to humans and South America's similar but separate species.

In 1950 the virus was introduced into rabbit warrens on the upper Murray River in Australia. At first nothing happened. Then, about 15 miles away, a sudden die-off of rabbits occurred. Soon the disease began to destroy the rabbit population in patches, sometimes making leaps of

100 miles at time. Ultimately the disease spread throughout Australia, moving most rapidly when moist conditions or standing water encouraged the mosquito vectors.

Despite a 99 percent initial mortality rate, the disease didn't kill all the rabbits. Within two years the virulence had declined to roughly 90 percent, and the rabbits survived longer after they got the disease. In time both the virus and the rabbits evolved. The disease's virulence declined—it killed only about 80 percent of those infected. And each year fewer and fewer rabbits got infected. At the start, practically all the rabbits were susceptible and got the disease. After six years, only about 30 percent were susceptible.

Eventually, the rabbits and the disease reached a rough equilibrium, the virus still highly lethal but with many rabbits unaffected. It did, however, kill 80 percent of the rabbit population in the process of reaching a stable relationship. It would not be surprising to discover that in a century's time it becomes as benign to the European species of rabbits as to their South American relatives. These same principles have long defined the relationship between microscopic predators and human beings.

CHAPTER THREE

AFTER THE GARDEN OF EDEN

Leaving the Garden of Eden might well have improved the lifespan of our earliest ancestors. As the earliest protohumans developed in the steamy rain forests of Africa more than five million years ago, they had no exclusive rights in the cradle of life. Instead, they must have clung to a small niche in a world densely populated by divergent evolutionary experiments in survival. This cornucopia of biological diversity included an exceptionally large and varied collection of predators of microscopic size. Such rain forests today harbor 20 different strains of malaria, and at least 150 different insect-borne viruses. A moist and invariably warm climate also supports an awesome array of fleas, ticks, mites, worms, protozoa, fungi and bacteria. So little evidence remains we can only guess when this began, and what a typical lifespan might have been. But for thousands of years these prehumans must have lived in a stable equilibrium with microscopic predators in great number. Then things began to change.

One primate species began hunting animals on the grassy plains of Africa, beginning a new contest for survival that provided rich rewards for intelligence, communication and teamwork. On the drier savannahs, many of the microscopic predators of the jungle could not survive. With a smaller burden of disease predation, the hunters and gatherers of the plains may well have been more vigorous than their evolutionary cousins who remained in the rain forest. But at the same time, new predators soon adapted to the two-legged creatures now prowling the vast plains of Africa. Surely one was a protozoan called the trypanosome, which infects the grazing animals of Africa. It is transported in the saliva glands of the tsetse fly and, when the fly bites, enters the bloodstream. No sooner does the human immune system identify and begin to neutralize this invader than the trypanosome changes its protein coat, appearing to the immune system to be a different organism. In laboratory experiments it has changed its immune profile 100 times, and may be able to do so 1,000 times. If the disease reaches the brain the result is a coma and death. The common name for this disorder is sleeping sickness, and to this day, it limits the number, lifespan and activities of men and animals over perhaps one-third of Africa.

Perhaps one million years ago, small groups of humans expanded into new territory armed with still another epochal innovation: clothing to protect them from adverse weather. From the cradle of life in Africa, and perhaps from Asia as well, humans began to spread rapidly over the globe, and by 10,000 years ago inhabited every continent except Antarctica. As humans moved into a colder climate they proliferated like the rabbits introduced into the alien ecology of Australia. There were fewer competitors for the food. Isolated human bands make a difficult target for diseases that don't have other animal victims. Some scholars who have examined this question with care, in particular William H. McNeill of the University of Chicago, conclude that the invigorating effects of the cooler weather were minor in comparison with the differences in disease predation. A huge share of Africa's microscopic predators of man simply couldn't survive in climates that were colder and drier. The fundamental, age-old equilibrium had been destroyed forever.

At a point reckoned 10,000 years before the present day, the first crude assessments of human life expectancy can be attempted. What was the starting point? After the first leap from a state of nature, what was the lifespan of humans in the Stone Age? What were the prospects for people who lived in caves and used simple stone tools? On the Maghreb Peninsula in Morocco are caves that sheltered Neolithic families for 1,500 years. A total of 186 skeletons survived. By Shigekazu Hishinuma's calculations, life expectancy at birth was just 15 years. The average length of life was so low because of an astronomical infant mortality rate. Those who survived to age 10 could expect to live, on the average, to 26.*

On Cyprus is a cemetery at least 5,000 years old. By Hishinuma's

---

*See notes for details of the basis of Hishinuma's and other calculations of early lifespans.

reckoning, life expectancy at birth was similar, about 16 years. But those who survived until age 10 appeared to live longer—perhaps into their early 30s. In Japan, the Jamon Age describes a 7,000-year period ending a few centuries before Christ. At the beginning of the Jamon Age, 10,000 years ago, the early Japanese people lived in pits dug into the mountainside and hunted, fished and collected plants. By the end of the period they sometimes farmed and built crude homes. From burial mounds in several locations in Japan, a total of 236 skeletons have been recovered. Life expectancy at birth was similar to that found in Cyprus and Morocco—about 16 years. Upon reaching age 10, an individual could expect to survive to the mid-20s. The life table estimates suggest that barely half those born would survive to reproductive age, or about 15. And only about 10 percent would ever live past age 30.

One of the great philosophical debates of all time concerns the virtues and character of man in a state of nature, compared with current times. In Christian and Moslem theology, the concept is expressed as the fall from the Garden of Eden. In secular philosophical terms, Rousseau described a noble savage corrupted by modern-day society. In the arena of health, a related idea surfaces in the advice that we should eat the diet of our primitive ancestors. This is one basis on which a diet low in salt and animal products is sometimes advocated. From the perspective of life expectancy, it seems foolish to model any practice on societies with a typical life expectancy of 15 or 16 years. Even if primitive man spent thousands of years adapting to a particular diet—a fact that is not certain—it need only sustain his health through a lifespan that was brutally short. If evolution favored any diet as mankind first expanded across the face of the globe, the advantage likely went to those who remained vigorous while consuming whatever food could be found, animal or vegetable.

For hundreds, even thousands of years, humans organized themselves into ever more advanced and complex societies with little apparent impact on life expectancy. The ancient Greeks wrote plays that are alive and meaningful 2,500 years later. Aristotle and Plato established fundamentals of social and political thought that endure unsurpassed to the present day. The Greeks emphasized a regimen of exercise, fresh air, and moderation in diet that might pass for acceptable health advice today. Hippocrates, for example, demonstrates a substantial grasp of health essentials:

"When one comes to a city . . . one ought to consider . . . the waters which the inhabitants use, whether they be marshy and soft or hard and running from elevated and rocky situations . . . whether it lies in a hollow and confined situation or is elevated and cold."

He also suggests examining the lifestyles of the residents: "Are they fond of drinking and eating to excess, and given to indolence, or are they fond of exercise and labor?"

The Greeks, however, also initiated a theory of disease causation that would mislead mankind for centuries. The human body was controlled by the four humors: blood, phlegm, yellow bile and black bile. The brain, in this doctrine, was the gland that secreted phlegm. Disease occurred because the humors got out of balance. Life expectancy in classical Greece cannot be measured accurately, but probably was only slightly better at birth than among Stone Age peoples: about 17 years. However, among those who survived to age 10 the prospects were better, with survival to the late 30s being typical.

In republican times, Rome boasted an abundant supply of clean water, and both public and private toilets that drained into a sewage system. Large and spacious public baths encouraged standards of personal cleanliness that would not be seen again in Europe for centuries. The Romans developed a centralized administration, a formidable military machine, and a network of roads that helped unify Europe and the Mediterranean world. But in the grasp of the threats of disease, they added only additional misconceptions to the erroneous Greek doctrine. The 22 volumes of Claudius Galen codified and expanded Roman medical knowledge and served as an authoritative text for the next one thousand years. But life expectancy improved little, if any, over that of the Greeks. One study of the epitaphs on 9,980 early Roman graves yields an average age at death of 22 years. When adjusted for the likely mortality of infants dying at or near birth without graves, Roman life expectancy appears comparable with the Greeks.

Medieval times were a disaster for civilization and for human life expectancy in Europe. The feudal Christian societies of Europe managed to discard the best of Roman and Greek doctrine (high standards of hygiene and sanitation) and retain the worst (the rigid and incorrect dogma about disease). Straitlaced early religious leaders frowned on bathing on moral grounds, and personal cleanliness didn't become part of Western culture until many centuries later. Queen Isabella of Spain is alleged to have boasted that she had taken only two baths in her entire life. Even in the American colonial era, lack of public baths or running water in homes meant bathing was a rarity.

The six centuries after the fall of Rome also brought the two greatest disease catastrophes in all of recorded history, and possibly the two greatest setbacks the human race has ever suffered. The more familiar of these disasters is the bubonic or black plague. Beginning on the shores of the Black Sea in 1346, the bubonic plague repeatedly swept through Europe during the fourteenth century. By the year 1400 it is likely that the population of Europe was reduced by 50 percent. Quarantine was the only defense of a society that did not understand how disease could be transmitted. And even that measure was ineffective because it did not control the rats that carried the fleas that harbored one of the most deadly bacteria that the world has ever known. It was a mysterious biological accident. Black rats invaded and occupied the growing cities of Europe. Thousands of miles away—on the plains of central Asia— plague-infected fleas leaped from rodent species who could tolerate the disease to the black rats, who could not. As the plague killed off the rats, the fleas desperately sought new hosts and settled on humans.

The second great disease catastrophe commands much less attention even though its causes are much better understood. As noted earlier, the animals, plants and peoples of North and South America were biologically isolated from Europe, Asia and Africa for thousands of years. When Europeans first made contact with the burgeoning, advanced civilizations of Mexico and Peru the result was an unprecedented biological tragedy.

The real reason a few hundred Spanish conquistadors could conquer the mighty Aztec empire was that they carried diseases to which the American natives had no immune defenses whatever. Within weeks of when Cortez landed in Mexico, smallpox was ravaging the Aztec civilization. Added to the actual toll of direct mortality was the psychological effect of a disease that killed so many of the leaders of the Aztec civilization while leaving the invaders untouched. Over a longer time, the

European diseases simply killed off the population. One authoritative estimate, for example, suggests a population of 25 million in Mexico and Central America in 1518. By 1568 the population had been reduced to 3 million; by 1620 it was cut in half again. A similarly drastic reduction in population occurred when Pizarro encountered the Incas of Peru. When the Pilgrims landed in Massachusetts in 1620, their tenuous hold in the New World was likely strengthened because 99 percent of the Massachusetts Indians had perished from disease in a massive epidemic two winters before. This was likely the outermost ripples of a wave of disease initiated when the Spanish first arrived in lower America. While Europe slowly recovered from the setbacks of disease in the fourteenth century, the great civilizations of the Americas were simply extinguished by smallpox, measles, yellow fever and typhus.

The evidence is less certain, but it is possible the American natives passed to European invaders a new and virulent strain of syphilis that killed quickly, unlike the modern variant. A syphilis epidemic first swept across Europe from Spain soon after the first voyages to the New World, but the evidence that it came from the Americas remains scanty.

For countless centuries, this was how humans shared the planet with microscopic life-forms, totally unaware of the true nature of the adversary that had regulated life expectancy since the Stone Age. The spectacular catastrophes may have been less important than the daily, weekly and monthly losses of talented human beings in the prime of vigorous life. The actual deaths may have been less important than how disease shaped the world view of a people who could be struck down by a mysterious force without warning, who watched hopelessly as disease claimed the lives of their spouses and young children.

The relationship between man and disease was never stable. Dreaded pestilence would arise and sweep through city after city, and then disappear. Other diseases—for example, the poorly understood "English sweats"—appeared, took their toll, and then disappeared forever. The increasing concentrations of people in cities provided new competitive advantage to those diseases that leaped from person to person. In the more sparsely settled countryside the most successful diseases needed an animal or insect vector. New possibilities were created when simple, but remarkably seaworthy sailing ships spanned the globe, bearing a cargo of new commerce, new ideas and new diseases.

. . .

By the year 1797 civilization had produced the *Iliad* of Homer and the military ideas of Julius Caesar; the ceiling of the Sistine Chapel bore Michelangelo's magnificent fresco; Mozart had completed 41 symphonies, and the human outlook had been enlarged by the dramatic visions of Milton, Voltaire and Shakespeare; Adam Smith had described the human transactions that increased and decreased "the wealth of nations"; Galileo, Copernicus and Kepler had reached toward infinity, expanding our knowledge of the heavens and explaining the principles by which whole planets move; Isaac Newton had formulated the mathematical laws that predict the movement of objects influenced by conflicting and invisible forces; the Dutch drapery merchant van Leeuwenhoek had reported finding tiny creatures of unknown purpose swimming in a drop of water; and in North America, thirteen former British colonies were testing a new blueprint for self-government. Perhaps more important than these isolated flashes of genius was a civilization that continuously preserved, passed on and developed the best that it had achieved.

Humans still had no clue to the relationship between mankind and microscopic forms of life, despite its being a subject of intense interest for more than 20 centuries. No one had a clear idea how disease moved from person to person, nor understood why some succumbed and others were spared. Humans were sharing a whole planet with a burgeoning world of sophisticated microscopic life with only meager clues to its very existence. These creatures inhabited their hands, rode on their skin, hid in their ears, multiplied in their digestive tracts, and no one knew anything about them.

As a consequence, human life expectancy had changed little. By the eighteenth century the first consistent birth and death records appear in a few cities, notably Vienna and Breslau, and genuine life tables can be constructed. Calculations from those records show life expectancy at birth had advanced from the 15 or 16 years in the Stone Age into the low 20s. By the end of the 1700s, some countries may have had life expectancies in the 30s. For survivors of the perils of birth and early childhood who reached age 10, the picture was brighter: on the average they could expect to reach age 60. But even these gains among adults may be exaggerated in the first calculations based on detailed systematic records rather than a few dozen skeletal remains.

Microscopic predators had been an invisible partner in human civilization for so many centuries that it was an epochal event when human beings first began to reshape this age-old relationship. On May 14, 1797, an English country doctor named Edward Jenner made a careful series of drawings of the sores that had appeared on the hands and wrists of Sarah Nelmes, the daughter of a local farmer. Then he pierced one of the sores with the tip of a medical lancet to obtain some of the infected matter. Using the same lancet, he made two scratches on the arm of James Phipps, age 8. Then he began to watch what, if anything, would happen. On the tenth day Phipps developed a single pustule on his arm; it scabbed over and became a scar. In time, most of the people in the world would have one like it.

Jenner had conducted the world's first successful vaccination, seeking to protect Phipps from one of the most dread diseases of his time—smallpox. To do so he had deliberately infected the young boy with a related but benign animal disease, cowpox. Seven weeks later he would put this fledgling technique to the acid test. He inoculated young Phipps with a potentially lethal dose of smallpox. Nothing happened. After a year's delay and just four more test subjects—one of whom soon died—Jenner announced his discovery to the world in a 75-page pamphlet which he published at his own expense.

Jenner had first learned of the protective powers of cowpox as a teenage apprentice to a physician 30 years earlier. In the meantime he had practiced medicine, formed two drinking clubs for medical cronies, and won modest fame in scientific circles with his study of birds, culminating in *The Natural History of the Cuckoo*. His findings on smallpox, needless to say, were of paramount importance.

Smallpox not only left many victims disfigured for life, but accounted for perhaps 10 percent of all deaths in Europe at the end of the eighteenth century. The only alternative means of protection was deliberate inoculation with the disease itself, a dangerous procedure with uncertain results. The brick-shaped virus was so contagious that, in one study, a hospital patient was infected by viral particles that arrived on air currents that had drifted out the open window of a victim quarantined in a room one floor below.

After only a brief controversy, the practice of vaccination was rapidly accepted around the world. It would be many decades before vaccination would be universal in entire countries, but its extraordinary value was immediately appreciated. It was hailed, quite appropriately, as the greatest discovery in the history of medicine. It also marked the coming of a global civilization capable of testing, reporting and then using widely a major scientific discovery about disease.

The coming of the first truly effective tool to prevent a deadly disease triggered a debate that would occur repeatedly as other threats to life were tamed. Would the elimination of a major killer like smallpox extend human life expectancy? Or would other death rates simply rise? One of the great pessimists of intellectual history, Thomas R. Malthus, thought vaccination would be pointless.

"I do not think that there has been produced any definite proofs that since the ancient times up to the present, the life of man has been prolonged," Malthus concluded. "Smallpox is in itself a pitfall which nature has provided in order to contain the population within bonds of living resources, and the pitfall is an extremely wide one. Either the pitfall will be made wider by nature, or else a new aperture will be created."

Malthus, writing at the dawn of the modern era, had grasped the fundamental forces that had long regulated both population size and life expectancy. He did not, however, realize the extent to which human beings were going to change this relationship. It is important, nevertheless, to retain perspective. To tout Jenner's achievement as an important part of the "conquest of disease" is somewhat like telling a man who has built the first wooden bridge over a tidewater pool that he has tamed the ocean.

In 1845 London was racked by the terrible pestilence of cholera. The year before it had erupted in India, and then swept toward the shores of the Caspian Sea. It killed more than 200,000 in Russia, and then rolled west toward Europe. By winter it had reached London. There, a young society doctor named John Snow was going to employ an entirely different kind of tool to combat disease. His substantial medical reputation in London had come because he was among the first British physicians to appreciate the possibilities of anesthesia, and would later attend Queen Victoria at the birth of her two children. In the meantime, Snow focused on one of the most deadly diseases of the time.

Cholera can trigger a diarrhea so violent that death occurs because the body has lost too much fluid to maintain blood pressure. Since it was a disorder of the intestinal tract, Snow concluded that whatever caused it must be somehow consumed by mouth. Given that it was a diarrheal condition, he grasped one of the most important of all vehicles for the transmission of disease: the fecal-oral route. Then, with good reason, his suspicions turned toward London's water supplies. The Southwark and Vauxhall Company's water intake was located on the Thames River just three yards from an outfall for raw sewage. On the other hand, another water company, Lambeth, had moved its intake well upriver from the city's sewage discharge points. The two companies competed for customers both rich and poor, and sometimes supplied adjacent buildings on the same street. Snow compared the two, producing a now famous table:

Water Company	Number of Houses	Cholera Deaths	Deaths per 10,000 Houses
Southwark & Vauxhall	40,046	1,263	315
Lambeth	26,107	98	37
Rest of London	256,423	1,442	59

It is one of the first systematic studies of the occurrence of disease, and marks a beginning point for the science of epidemiology. Do those affected share some common factor—in this case drinking water from a certain source—that will lead us to the actual cause or the means to prevent disease?

While epidemiology offers one of the most important of all tools for understanding health and longevity, it also introduces a great dilemma. What is convincing evidence? The statistical association that Snow observed is quite different from the direct causal chain that Jenner demonstrated. There was no question that young Phipps was protected from smallpox. Jenner inoculated him directly with the disease to prove it.

But take a deep drink of Southwark's contaminated water and probably nothing will happen. Invite a hundred neighbors to share in this repast. The result will likely be the same—or perhaps a single case.

Epidemiology depends on the fascinating but inherently slippery business of inferences and associations. True, the Southwark and Vauxhall's customers were 10 times more likely to get cholera than Lambeth's. But how does Snow explain why at least 97 percent of Southwark's customers were still free of disease? How many victims were exposed to the disease in a manner that Snow overlooked? Today we know cholera can also be transmitted by personal contact, be carried by flies, be contracted through seafood, and be passed by contamination of clothes, cooking utensils and food.

Snow's complete inquiry into the causes of cholera, published in 1855, provided something to satisfy the conflicting views of the proper role of epidemiology. Those who fear that such statistical associations may frequently mislead us about health threats honor the thoroughness of Snow's overall investigation. He conducted a lengthy series of experiments, the water company comparison being just one. Those with a more enthusiastic opinion of epidemiology see something entirely different in Snow's work. They argue that Snow's systematic analysis revealed how cholera was transmitted 31 years before germ theory was conclusively established. To this faction, the lure of epidemiology is the potential capacity to attack health problems in which the disease process remains unknown. As later chapters will show, the epidemiological dilemma that began 150 years ago runs deeply through modern-day research about diet, exercise, obesity, cancer and heart disease.

Interestingly, the most important contributions to human life expectancy in the 1850s were made by people who thought John Snow was dead wrong about cholera. In London, Munich, Boston and New York, public-spirited individuals were crusading with substantial effectiveness against "filth."

Attention to the problem was long overdue. Bathing was rare. Drinking water was often polluted. The streets were filled with garbage and excrement from humans and horses. The burgeoning cities of the industrial revolution were overcrowded by an appalling mass of hungry, filthy, vermin-infested humanity.

The sworn enemies of filth promoted clean water, sewage systems, ventilation and fresh air as healthy in their own right. Many proponents of this approach, including Florence Nightingale and Munich's Max von Pettenkofer, vigorously resisted the idea of person-to-person contagion through germs. They argued it undermined the importance of a healthy environment in preventing disease. You avoided disease, in this view, by fresh air and healthy living, not because you happened to touch the wrong person. This led to an often unfocused attack that addressed sources of filth—for example, the stench of tanneries—that had little or nothing to do with disease.

Did the mid-eighteenth century opponents of germ theory do humanity a great disservice by defending for 30 years the doctrine that disease could be caused by an invisible miasma in the air? Might we all be much farther along the rising curve of human longevity without such a lengthy debate and delay? A similar issue arises today with enthusiastic accounts of promising but not completely proven new drugs and other approaches to improving health or extending life. Regularly, the Food and Drug Administration is criticized for demanding lengthy additional experiments and testing. Is it a service to humanity or an unnecessary delay in progress to demand full, complete and convincing proof? Oddly enough, the germ theory debate provides a compelling answer to that question.

By the 1850s the acquisition of new knowledge no longer depended on the sporadic but earthshaking revelations of an English country doctor or a Dutch drapery merchant with a hobby of grinding microscope lenses. The scientific method was in full flower. It offered much more than an approach under which the experimenter stated a hypothesis and identified the evidence that proved or disproved it. The truly compelling power of the scientific method was that experiments were openly published, the results shared and vigorously debated. The opponents of germ theory were not blindly hewing to historical dogma. They loosed a torrent of perfectly logical objections and performed convincing experiments.

One of the most famous such demonstrations was offered by Max von Pettenkofer, whose public health crusades had brought a revolution in sanitation to Munich. The legendary German microbiologist Robert Koch had announced he had discovered the bacteria that caused cholera, after identifying it in the water supply of Calcutta. Furthermore, he had an explanation why it did not invariably cause disease. The cholera bacillus is sensitive to acid, and in some circumstances may be killed by the hydrochloric acid secreted in the stomach.

Von Pettenkofer conceded the bacillus was involved in the disease, but maintained the bacteria were of little importance without other environmental factors. He offered to prove his point. After taking a large dose of sodium carbonate to neutralize stomach acid, he swallowed large numbers of cholera bacteria recently cultured from a fatal case. There were no consequences except a case of light diarrhea.

The germ theory debate had one far-reaching consequence: By the time that Robert Koch, Louis Pasteur, Joseph Lister and other pioneers of microbiology emerged victorious they had not simply proven the validity an interesting theory. They had mastered the fundamentals of the bacterial world. They could grow different kinds of bacteria in pure culture. They found species that were killed by oxygen, bacteria that died without it, and switch hitters that changed when oxygen was available. The bacteria were heated, cooled, passed through filters and different species of animals. They were tested with acids, salts, sugar and alcohol.

It was an hour of great glory for the scientific method. Because the researchers openly published their results, one experimenter quickly spawned a new discovery by another. In Glasgow, Joseph Lister read of Pasteur's experiments in the fermentation of wine, which demonstrated that bacteria are nearly universally present floating in the air. It dawned on him that it was these organisms that were infecting wounds and surgical incisions. The idea of antisepsis was thus born.

In Germany, Robert Koch read about C. J. Davinine's inconclusive experiments in France suggesting that a rod-shaped bacterium might cause anthrax. In one of the most famous experiments in the history of science, Koch grew the anthrax bacillus in pure culture and caused disease at will by inoculating animals with the organisms, offering the decisive proof of germ theory.

Pasteur converted Koch's compelling but limited scientific proof into one of the most dazzling discoveries in all history. He was resuming experiments with chicken cholera in the fall of 1879 when he discovered that the cholera bacteria cultures he had kept over the summer no longer killed the chickens. When he inoculated them with the disease, nothing happened. From a recent outbreak, he obtained a fresh, virulent supply of bacteria. Then he inoculated a group of chickens again. Instead of killing all the chickens as expected, it killed only half of them.

A lesser mind might have discarded the stubborn chickens that did not die as germ theory so neatly predicted. A Louis Pasteur grasped the idea of acquired immunity. The chickens that died were newcomers to his lab, recently obtained from the market. The survivors had all been previously inoculated with the culture that had lost its potency. The bacteria had been weakened enough so that they didn't make the chickens sick, but the chickens were still made resistant to direct inoculation with fully virulent bacteria. He immediately made the connection to Edward Jenner's cowpox inoculation, and grasped the principle underlying all vaccination. If the human body was exposed to a specimen of a disease that had somehow been rendered incapable of causing harm, it would nevertheless learn how to repel the microscopic invader should it later arrive in fully virulent form.

Within a few years of Koch's demonstration that bacteria caused anthrax in sheep, Pasteur agreed to satisfy skeptics with a dramatic experiment: He would demonstrate how to protect the sheep from anthrax. In the legendary public trial, 24 vaccinated sheep, 1 goat and 6 cows remained healthy even when inoculated with the disease; an equal number of unvaccinated animals died, 2 of which obediently dropped dead before the spectators who had arrived to observe the experiment's outcome. Later experimenters, with many years of experience with unpredictable clinical trials, would say privately that not only was Pastuer exceptionally bold, he was unusually lucky that nothing unexpected happened to wreck the experiment. The achievement was still no less impressive. Jenner had mastered a technique that happened to work. Pasteur had established a concept that would now begin to protect all mankind from its predators. Now, for the first time in history, it was possible to set forth in a planned, deliberate way to alter the age-old balance with microscopic life-forms.

At the dawn of the twentieth century, the breathtaking discoveries of Pasteur, Koch and Lister had given way to new lessons in humility. Humans could be protected from smallpox, and farm animals from anthrax. Heat milk briefly, and it killed most of the microorganisms living therein. Clean up the drinking water, and the cholera and typhoid fever cases would decline dramatically. Pasteur had shown how to build immunity to rabies, but rabies was extremely rare.

On the other hand, pneumonia killed people every day. No longer was there any doubt what caused it. Usually, the pneumococcus bacteria could be readily identified in the respiratory tract of those afflicted with an unproductive cough and a soaring fever. In a shocking number of cases, perhaps one out of three, young healthy patients simply died and there was little anybody could do.

Lister's antiseptics had contributed greatly to reducing the incidence of wound infection, but understandably infections still occurred with great frequency. However, better-controlled experiments showed that pouring antiseptic chemicals into an open infected wound did more harm than good. Some of the bacteria were killed. But the antiseptic never reached others. It also killed the white blood cells that were eating the bacteria; in fact, it was somewhat more effective against the white blood cells than against the hardier bacteria.

Sometimes technical difficulties provided a roadblock. It was extremely difficult to grow some microscopic organisms in a laboratory. If you couldn't grow them, how could you study them? Finally, there were agents that could be neither grown nor seen. They were called filterable viruses because they were so tiny they passed through fine porcelain filters that captured all bacteria.

It is therefore not surprising that a German physician and chemist named Paul Ehrlich should yearn for a magic bullet to slay the large majority of microscopic invaders that still eluded the grasp of science.

As any beginning biology student learns, it is in fact difficult to see any kind of cell under a microscope without stains. Stains, of course, are chemical dyes. And dyes are prominent among the chemicals with selective effects on cells. Methylene blue stains nerve cells but not the adjacent tissue. Bacteria are classified as Gram-negative or Gram-positive according to whether they become visible under a microscope when stained with Christian Gram's chemical dye. If Ehrlich was going to devote years to the search for a magic bullet, he wanted to see what was happening. So he focused on dyes.

Ehrlich's idea was a conceptual breakthrough of a new kind. He didn't have a magic bullet. He theorized that it was reasonable that there be such a chemical, announced the idea publicly, and set forth systematically to search for one. He never really succeeded. The closest he came was more like a biological hammer than a magic bullet. It was a chemical relative of arsenic that killed off the syphilis spirochete somewhat quicker than it did the patient. His most powerful contribution was a concept, an entirely new way of thinking about how to deal with microscopic predators that breach the body defenses: try to find something that will kill them without also dispatching their prey.

More than 20 years later Gerhard Domagk, a German chemist, was following Ehrlich's prescription, and routinely screening the dyes developed by the chemical giant I. G. Farben. In 1932 he tested a new product called Prontosil, which produced in textiles a lovely rich gold hue. Had he been following the lab protocols used in England or America he would have placed some of the chemical in a petri dish with a culture of bacteria and observed what happened. Had he done so, it would have been on to the next chemical. But German company regulations required that each new chemical be routinely tested for biological effects in live animals. When injected into mice, it attacked streptococcus bacteria, while having little or no effect on the mouse. French researchers quickly confirmed Domagk's work, adding an additional revelation. Prontosil was quickly broken down in the body to the more commonplace chemical sulfanilamide. This chemical had been well characterized in 1908 by an Austrian printing-ink chemist.

The drug that was selective for bacteria had an electric effect on biological thinking around the world. It meant there had to be even better ones. At Rockefeller University, a bacteriologist named Rene Dubos concluded that the search ought to be conducted, not in a man-made chemical factory, but in the greatest chemical factory in the world, in nature. In 1939 he found a soil bacteria, *Bacillus brevis,* that synthesized a substance that broke apart pneumonia and streptococcus bacteria. Like Ehrlich's first discovery, Dubos's natural antibiotic was also quite toxic to humans, and had limited use. Dubos, however, thought that someone ought to take a close look at Alexander Fleming's mold juice, which had been a laboratory curiosity since 1928. When two Oxford pathologists did exactly that, they documented the wonders of penicillin in one year's time.

It still might have been of little medical importance. An obscure mold did fabricate a unique organic molecule that prevents a wide variety of bacteria from creating its tough sugar coat at cell division. Since no human cells require this external skeleton, it was remarkably nontoxic. But where do you get millions of gallons of this exotic compound? Fleming, in fact, had abandoned his experiments with penicillin when two assistants had labored for a year without success to produce penicillin in enough quantity to continue an experimental program. The real breakthrough at Oxford was a better approach to getting the stuff; testing it was easy. But still they produced only experimental quantities. In one of those extraordinary feats of wartime cooperation, a U.S. Department of Agriculture lab in Peoria and five drug companies quickly learned how to grow the strange mold in industrial quantities.

An extraordinary transformation in thinking about the microscopic world had been completed. The hardest part was simply understanding how to approach the problem. Bacteria had been known for three centuries before Koch demonstrated to the satisfaction of all that they caused disease. But even knowledge was not enough. It was necessary for only a relatively small number of scientists and engineers to have mastered Isaac Newton's laws of motion. Changing the human species' relationship to disease required cooperative action on a massive scale, whether the issue was vaccination, sanitation or mustering resources to produce and purify enormous quantities of a compound secreted by an obscure species of mold. Reflecting on the overall story, one is left with a dual sense of wonder: surprise that it took so long to discover a relationship so basic and amazement at how swiftly and forcefully the industrialized world acted once it understood.

CHAPTER FOUR

THE GREAT LONGEVITY GAIN

There are disturbing inconsistencies in the conventional explanations of why life expectancy has steadily increased in the United States and Europe over a long period. For example, we are told to credit better sanitation and the elimination of contaminated water and food; but the most important changes occurred among respiratory diseases that could not have been much affected by these measures. Was it better nutrition? Since 1900 there has been plenty of protein, fat and calories in the American diet, and in recent years perhaps an excess. At the same time, life expectancy increased by 34 years. Others credit the conquest of the childhood diseases of diphtheria, whooping cough and scarlet fever; but all three had mostly disappeared before effective immunization programs were in operation. Examined carefully, the conventional wisdom does not stand up.

A lengthy period of steady gains produces a special challenge to analysis because simultaneous improvements occurred in many potential factors: income, housing, job and public safety, medical treatment, immunization, maternal health, infant mortality and sanitation. Without simply indulging one's favorite cause, how does one identify which factor properly deserves credit? Despite the pitfalls, this is an effort worth undertaking. Bringing the causes of the century-and-a-half gain into a reasoned perspective will reveal the main sources of current successes and lay the foundation for examining the prospects for future gains.

This is of far more than academic interest. Emphasizing the wrong reasons for the great gain in human life expectancy will lead to misguided policies to obtain future gains. At best this wastes time and money better devoted to achieving improvements; at worst it risks losing ground already gained. This might come in a cataclysmic new killer plague that should have been anticipated, or might occur as much more subtle and difficult-to-detect losses in health status.

It is hard to identify a specific point when, after centuries without major improvement, life expectancy began to improve steadily year after year. The sustained trend probably began around 1750, certainly by 1800. By the year 1841, when the oldest continuous chain of evidence begins, life expectancy had already exceeded 40 years. That is already an impressive increase from the previous century, when fragmentary information suggests life expectancy ranged from the low 20s to the low 30s.

Beginning in 1800, smallpox vaccination began to have an effect, but could not conceivably have produced a gain of more than 10 years so quickly. In some of the countries with the earliest health records—for example, Sweden—the evidence suggests even smallpox deaths had already declined dramatically before vaccination was introduced, a pattern observed repeatedly with other diseases.

So, unfortunately, it is necessary to begin without an important piece of the puzzle—an understanding of what produced the first important gains in life expectancy. So sketchy is the surviving evidence the answer must necessarily be left in the shadows of imperfectly recorded history. The productive search, therefore, begins in England about 1840, the earliest date at which comprehensive birth and cause-of-death information becomes available. (In the United States, similar information for select states does not begin until 1900.)

One approach to unraveling the secrets of the great gain in life expectancy is to ask the simple questions first. Were there major perils to life in 1841 that have become unimportant today? For an answer, one need look no further than the most important cause of death in 1841, and one of the greatest killers of all time—the disease tuberculosis.

Once it defined how millions of young men and women lived and died, how they thought about themselves and their world. At the apex of its power and virulence, tuberculosis was a terror of such magnitude there is no modern-day counterpart. Would American history be different if TB had not killed George Washington's capable older brother,

Lawrence, who outshone his younger sibling as a political and military leader until his early death? What effect did a continuous low-grade fever have on Thoreau's perceptions at Walden Pond? Would the English novel have reached the same heights if TB had not killed Charlotte and Emily Bronte's two younger sisters? TB killed the poet Keats. Shelley drowned while seeking treatment in Italy. It claimed Chopin and helped end the life of the most renowned violinist of all time, Nicolo Paganini. Cecil Rhodes made a fortune and founded a white empire in South Africa while seeking a hot dry climate for his tuberculosis. It struck the ordinary and the famous, the rich and poor. Telltale evidence of tuberculosis can be found among the skeletal remains of Stone Age families, but it probably reached a peak among the dirty, crowded cities of the industrial revolution. No region, no city, no neighborhood was untouched, and rare was the family that escaped.

The many separate faces of tuberculosis were not recognized as effects of the same disease until quite late. Tuberculosis of the lung has been well known at least since the ancient Greeks named it phthisis. But for centuries no connection was made to tubercular infection of the lymph nodes of the neck, then believed to be a separate disease called scrofula. When TB invaded the bones, it often produced the distinctive curved spine of the Hunchback of Notre Dame. While usually a slow, wasting disease lasting many years, a runaway tuberculous infection called "the galloping consumption" could claim its victim within days.

Prior to the germ theory era, the desperate search for an effective treatment led to some of the most foolish attempted cures in the annals of medicine. Some prescribed the invigorating fumes of cow manure; others suggested horseback riding or saxophone playing. Those without the funds for an extended ocean voyage could purchase a special mechanical chair whose movements were intended to induce the nausea often encountered on a rough sea passage. The touch of a king or queen was believed to cure the swollen lymph nodes of scrofula. There were proponents of hot climates and cold breezes, of dry desert air and the moist atmosphere of the seaside.

Imagine, then, the excitement triggered in 1892 when one of the most famous medical men in the world, Robert Koch, announced that he had found a cure for tuberculosis. Ten years earlier, Koch had identified beyond doubt the causative organism, *Mycobacterium tuberculo-*

sis. It was an extremely slow-growing bacterium with an unusual waxy outer protein coat. While typical bacteria divided in less than an hour, *Mycobacterium tuberculosis* did so only once or twice every day. Needless to say, Koch's announcement was greeted by worldwide rejoicing.

A. Conan Doyle, the British doctor-author whose most famous effort was the legendary fictional detective Sherlock Holmes, traveled to Germany to investigate and report on the momentous discovery. But demonstrating some of the powers of observation for which Holmes was famous, Doyle expressed skepticism about Koch's discovery. What Koch had really found, Doyle concluded, might be very valuable but was not, in fact, the long-sought cure. Koch had isolated a distinctive protein manufactured by the tuberculosis bacteria. An immune system response to this alien protein became the basis for the tuberculin test, but it did not create immunity, as Koch had hoped. Nevertheless here was an important tool to identify those who might be harboring this disease without knowing it.

Soon the newly developed tuberculin test was used in several major cities to measure the extent of the disease. The results were a tremendous shock. Practically everyone showed evidence of infection—young and old, the vigorous and ailing, those with symptoms and those without the slightest evidence of disease. This was not how germ theory was supposed to work! Infection occurred when bacteria were transmitted from one person to the next, particularly in the air, water or food. If nearly everyone was infected with the disease, why were some not affected? What separated those who remained healthy from those who slowly wasted away, dying a painful death as the bacteria destroyed ever-increasing amounts of vital lung tissue? It was a sobering introduction to one complexity of man's relationship with infectious disease. Furthermore, it is clear that better sewage systems and an uncontaminated water supply may have had a large impact on cholera and other intestinal diseases transmitted through the fecal-oral route, but these factors had little or no impact on respiratory bacteria moving from person to person through the air.

Thus no cure was available in 1892 or for many decades thereafter. Not until 1946 was a drug discovered to eliminate an active tuberculosis infection. And even then it took a six-month course of treatment with an antibiotic called streptomycin.

Now comes the chapter in the story of the conquest of disease that is often omitted from conventional accounts. By the time an effective cure was finally available, tuberculosis was no longer a major threat. So what had happened? Tuberculosis simply killed all those human beings who could not resist it. The whole process took perhaps 150 years in all, but exactly paralleled the fate of the rabbits in Australia that were infected with myxomatosis. If introduced into isolated human populations without any previous exposure, tuberculosis quickly killed a majority in the form of galloping consumption; a minority were spared and others suffered from a slowly advancing infection. In time, the toll of the disease slowly and steadily moderated.

Mankind conquered this disease the hard way, not through miracle drugs, but by the elimination of those unable to resist. Approximately 85 percent of the decline in tuberculosis occurred before the discovery of an effective treatment. While the gradual disappearance of tuberculosis falls well short of explaining the entire gain in life expectancy since 1841, it is the largest single contributor.

Tuberculosis has not completely disappeared today. Like the bubonic plague, it is simply lurking in the background. Consider a 1991 study of 543 North Carolina migrant workers, who share crowded, substandard living conditions and below-average health status. A total of 53 percent tested positive for tuberculosis. Only 2 percent, however, had clinically active disease. Not surprisingly, TB is also frequently seen in AIDS patients, and among recent emigrants from impoverished areas. In addition to being on the increase, TB is increasingly resistant to drugs now used to combat it. The Centers for Disease Control reported in 1991 the case of a former drug user with AIDS admitted to a Muskegon, Michigan, treatment facility for substance abuse. He proved to have TB resistant to three of the front-line drugs: isoniazid, rifampin and ethambutol. He also passed the resistant strain to at least 15 and possibly 22 other persons at the facility. In early 1992, health authorities became greatly concerned about the rapid spread of the resistant strain among those with compromised immune systems. Microscopic life forms adapt to any weakness in the defenses of human society.

Tuberculosis had an important rival as a peril to life in the previous century, another respiratory disease that was unlikely to be neutralized by personal hygiene or sanitation measures. The disease, pneumonia, remains a threat today, although hardly in such terrifying form. Pneumonia was so important in 1901 that when William Osler wrote one of the most famous medical textbooks in history, he described it as "Captain of All Men of Death."

A typical pneumonia case begins with nothing more ominous than the symptoms of a common cold. In the process, *Streptococcus pneumoniae* bacteria, which may have been harmlessly occupying the nasal cavity, become established in a lobe of one of the lungs and begin to multiply rapidly. The secret of its success—and principal source of its menace—can be found in its outer protein coat. It is so tough that the large white blood cells, called phagocytes, that are dispatched to engulf the pneumonia bacteria cannot destroy them. As a result, dead white blood cells, fluid and proliferating bacteria accumulate in great quantity in the affected area of the lung. This increases the weight of the lung by three to five times and triggers a running fever of 102–106 degrees F, a rapid heartbeat and often a sense of suffocating. The fever lasts for days, and before antibiotics, killed about one out of three who suffered a major, runaway infection. The fever finally broke only when the body began to manufacture large quantities of antibodies and the full defenses of the immune system were brought to bear. Victims were of all ages, but often young and healthy adults. If the patient was hardy enough to survive the sudden illness, there was usually no permanent damage to the lung.

Pneumonia was so common and so deadly that developing a vaccine became a priority early in the germ theory era. It proved to be enormously more difficult than expected. Antibodies that seek out invading bacteria are extremely specific—often attaching to a specific site of only one or two molecules. *S. pneumoniae* has a protein coat that varies just enough to require 84 different antibodies to provide immunity against all the subtypes.

Although tuberculosis began to wane before 1800, pneumonia did not enter a period of rapid decline until a century later, about 1900. It is also harder to track its decline accurately because pneumonia deaths are grouped with influenza, bronchitis and lung infections from other bacteria and from viruses. The best estimates suggest that about two-thirds of the decline in pneumonia occurred before effective treatment was available—the first sulfa drugs in 1935 and antibiotics in 1941. It is not clear why pneumonia initially declined. It might have been a by-product of the population's growing capacity to resist tuberculosis, or part of an improved general health status that, as we shall see, was apparently responsible for the decline of several other infectious diseases.

Today pneumonia remains an important cause of mortality, ranked sixth in the United States. Pneumonia now occurs primarily among the elderly and those with compromised immune systems. Even in the antibiotic era, pneumonia has a sobering 5 percent case fatality rate. So while it is less dangerous today, the bacteria are still found everywhere. For example, from 75 to 95 percent of all children experience infections of the middle ear—usually caused by *S. pneumoniae.*

The late British medical sociologist Thomas McKeown was among the first to observe that most of the decline in the big respiratory diseases—TB and pneumonia—could not properly be attributed to advances in medical care. His conclusion, in a book called *The Role of Medicine,* triggered an immediate controversy because his analysis of the gains in life expectancy in England gave medical care a relatively modest role. The medical world has been accustomed to taking virtually all the credit. Nevertheless, McKeown's careful and systematic examination of British mortality data has stood the test of time, and provides important insights into why life expectancy has steadily increased. His findings are ex-pressed in terms of death rates, rather than as years of life expectancy, but the effect is exactly the same.

McKeown found that roughly 40 percent of the reduction in mortal-ity since 1841 can be attributed to the decline, mostly spontaneous, in diseases transmitted by the respiratory route. While TB and pneumonia dominated the picture, there were similar reductions in other respiratory diseases. For example, measles was once a lethal childhood disease. Until an immunization campaign began in 1963, it remained among the most common diseases. But the virulence of the disease declined steadily for over 100 years to reach such low levels that case fatality rates were not even routinely published by the time the immunization campaign was launched to eradicate it. By contrast, however, when the Australians accidentally introduced measles to the completely unadapted Fiji Islanders in 1875, it killed 10 to 20 percent of the island population. Scarlet fever, diphtheria and whooping cough also became progressively less deadly year by year.

The most interesting of McKeown's findings lay in his calculations of how much immunization or other direct medical intervention contributed. He found 84 percent of the decline in TB came before effective treatment was developed; for pneumonia 68 percent of the drop preceded treatment; for whooping cough 90 percent; for scarlet fever and diphtheria, at least 70 percent. Thus, the largest share of the great gain in human life expectancy can be attributed to the continuous process of mutual adjustment between humans and microscopic life-forms. Direct benefits from the discoveries of the golden age of microbiology contributed less and came much later than commonly supposed.

Did the diseases become less virulent, or did humans grow better able to resist them? In the case of respiratory tuberculosis the picture is particularly clear that the disease ruthlessly destroyed a substantial fraction of mankind unable to resist it. The many episodes in which isolated populations were devastated by otherwise "benign" diseases suggest most adaptation occurred among human prey rather than microscopic predator. The methods for measuring virulence are so recent and primitive that few documented examples exist of independent changes in disease virulence. Among the respiratory killers, scarlet fever, which declined with unusual speed, is a leading suspect for having mutated into a more benign form.

Deliberate human intervention contributed much more to the parallel decline of diseases of the intestinal tract. McKeown attributes nearly 11 percent of the overall decline in the death rate in England to a reduction in cholera, and another 11 percent to other diseases of the intestinal tract. Although clear and concise data are lacking, there is no reason to challenge conventional assumptions that improvements in water, sewage, personal hygiene and food supplies are primarily responsible. Two qualifications are worthy of note. Modern-day efforts in Bangladesh have demonstrated that cholera cannot be prevented simply by providing uncontaminated fresh water. In the impoverished areas of Bangladesh, there proved to be so many sources of fecal contamination that a massive program to provide clean water wells had little effect. Secondly, a generally healthier population was better able to resist gastrointestinal disease even when confronted with contaminated food or water.

Additional insights into the great gain in life expectancy come from another landmark study. The eminent demographer Samuel Preston and two colleagues created detailed life expectancy tables for 42 nations over periods ranging from 1 to 104 years. The study included an enormous range of life expectancies, from 26 years (for Taiwanese males in 1920) to 76 years among Norwegian women in 1964. Then Preston combined all the observations into a massive statistical model to identify the differences among the countries with short, long and average lifespans.

Over a long period, in diverse countries and under quite different economic circumstances, Preston's data show one overwhelming influence: infectious disease defines the difference between nations with long and short life expectancies. Like McKeown, he ranks changes in the respiratory diseases as of primary importance. But in Preston's sample, which includes many tropical countries, intestinal diseases play a bigger role.

Perhaps the most concise illustration of the determinative factors and the limits of our current life expectancy can be found in a single table. Imagine a magic wand that would completely eliminate a particular cause of death, as immunization in fact achieved with smallpox and polio, or sanitation accomplishes with cholera. Then observe how it affects overall life expectancy.

Here are Preston's results, first for a semideveloped country such as England in 1850, Japan in 1900, or Chile in 1940.

FEMALES IN A SOCIETY WITH LIFE EXPECTANCY OF 40 YEARS	
Cause of Death Eliminated	Additional Lifespan
Violence & accidents	6 months
Cancer	9 months
Infectious disease	19 years

At more modern levels of life expectancy, however, the gains from infectious disease have been nearly exhausted. Also, this model illustrates

the limited potential of additional changes in any of the major causes of
death.

FEMALES IN A SOCIETY WITH LIFE EXPECTANCY OF 72 YEARS

Cause of Death Eliminated	Additional Lifespan
Violence & accidents	8 months
Cancer	2.5 years
Infectious disease	1.7 years

There are troubling implications from this overall body of evidence.
If hygiene, sanitation, immunization and direct medical interventions
explain only a fraction of the decline of infectious disease, why do people
become less vulnerable to TB, pneumonia, bronchitis and intestinal
disorders? Modern-day American physicians armed with antibiotics
could have effectively combated an acute case of pneumonia in one of
the otherwise healthy young women admitted to hospitals with pneumonia at the turn of the century. But such cases are extremely rare today.
Travelers suffer digestive disorders in less-developed countries where
sanitation is poor. But rarely are they fatal. Testing positive for TB is still
a fairly commonplace event; active disease is seldom found. What accounts for today's healthier, more robust specimens of the human species?

At this juncture many an otherwise careful analyst leaps blindly into
the last remaining conventional explanation: it must be better nutrition
that's making us live longer. In this instance the evidence is less clear, but
like the factors discussed above the role of nutrition is routinely exaggerated. The contribution of nutrition can be examined within the
framework of consumption patterns in the United States since 1910,
when life expectancy was just 49 years for men and 53 years for women.

The first question is simply, was there enough to eat? Modern healthy
human beings need less than 3,000 calories per day. Most think the
United States consumes too much at current levels of 3,600 calories a
day.* The long-lived Japanese consume 2,800 calories a day. In nations
where malnutrition is commonplace—for example, Somalia or the

---

*These national figures are based on food supply and are crude measures of amounts
actually consumed. They overstate human needs and omit, among other things, wast-
age. But unfortunately this is how food supply data are reported.

Sudan—total calories may range from 1,500 to 2,000 per day. By the time of the first published United States figures in 1909, more than 3,500 calories per person were available. The lowest figure was in 1960, still a generous 3,100 calories. There is no question that malnutrition shortens life expectancy, more often by increasing vulnerability to disease than from outright starvation. But in terms of total quantities available, there has been a plentiful supply in the United States during this century.

We also need plenty of protein. The body uses the 20 amino acids to fabricate an astonishing variety of essential substances. The body cannot manufacture 8 of these amino acids, and the precise balance needed is found in beef, pork and poultry, although they can also be obtained from a purely vegetarian diet with careful attention to detail. Since 1909 there has been more than 90 grams of protein a day in the U.S. diet. This amounts to roughly two times basic nutritional needs. The other major nutrient, fats, has been available in even more abundant quantities than calories or protein. Beyond quite small quantities of two essential fatty acids, the primary function of animal and vegetable fat is to enhance the taste of food and to provide calories in a form digested more slowly than carbohydrates. Over time, there have been changes, but not of an earthshaking character. At the turn of the century, lard rendered from animal fat was the primary cooking oil. Today most comes from vegetable sources. Americans have increasingly switched from butter to margarine, but the total amount of animal fat in the diet has remained fairly constant. Total calories and quantities of vegetable fat have risen.

It would be easier to credit nutrition for twentieth-century gains in longevity if either gradually or suddenly the United States had solved a long-term food supply problem. This did occur when some Asian nations introduced new rice hybrids creating a green revolution in food supply. But food has been plentiful and increasingly cheap through most of the United States' history.

Lack of specific nutrients can also shorten life substantially. Lack of vitamin C causes scurvy; not enough niacin results in pellagra. Beriberi and rickets result from vitamin deficiencies, but these diseases seldom occur in the absence of gross malnutrition. Scurvy is seen only under extreme conditions, such as the early sea voyages when the crew subsisted for months on hard tack. But these deficiencies produce severe and identifiable symptoms and cannot have been an important source of overall mortality in the United States in the twentieth century. Because the American diet has long featured large quantities of meat and milk, it is also unlikely that iron, calcium or potassium deficiencies were an issue.

It can be sensibly argued that the food problem in the United States was never the total supply, but that large numbers of the poor never got enough. Poor people have unquestionably suffered from genuine malnutrition. However, if we confine the analysis to groups that were unmistakably prosperous enough to eat adequately—for example, white males buying life insurance policies or the British nobility—we observe the same patterns of infectious disease receding at about the same rate. For a variety of reasons, nutrition likely counting among them, the prosperous live longer than average, and the impoverished shorter than average. However, both groups are subject to the same broad trends in longevity.

There are examples where nutrition and longevity are unmistakably intertwined. The most dramatic case was in Ireland, where peasants had enthusiastically embraced the New World's potato as the primary crop. The chief appeal was that an acre of land planted in potatoes supported fully twice as many people as an acre of wheat. When the potato blight destroyed Ireland's crop for two successive seasons in 1846–47, the results were catastrophic. Almost half the Irish population died or migrated. The direct causes of death were usually typhus and other diseases sweeping through the weakened population. England, which was not so dependent on the potato, suffered no famine, but scurvy occurred because potatoes and other succulent vegetables were scarce. The farther one pushes back before 1800 in Europe, the more likely that famine was a contributor to limits on life expectancy. It is undoubtedly a factor today in the impoverished nations of the horn of Africa. But it is unlikely nutrition had much effect on the rapid gains in life expectancy recorded in England and the United States beginning about 1880.

This argument occurred to another careful observer of long-term trends in longevity, a Palo Alto, California, physician and epidemiologist named Leonard Sagan. His crisply argued book, *The Health of Nations,* suggests that the real revolution in longevity occurred because of changes in infant mortality and early childhood care. As was noted earlier, the gains in life expectancy have not been distributed evenly across all ages.

The most dramatic changes occurred in infancy and early childhood. For example, in England 31 percent of all newborns died before age 10 in the year 1861. In the United States and Britain today 98.6 percent survive to age 10.

Sagan argues that this was more than a change in health status and the burden of disease; this was a change in attitude. Once some threshold in the chance of infant survival is surpassed, parents begin to cherish their children. When and where this occurs, survival rates improve dramatically, and overall life expectancy grows rapidly.

A large body of evidence—ranging from the crusading fiction of Charles Dickens to the pamphlets of English reformers—documents the murder, neglect, abandonment and mistreatment of infants and children in the preceding century. In addition, Sagan chronicles other disastrous child-rearing practices—premature weaning, overworked wet nurses and grossly contaminated food—that sharply reduced survival rates. The benefits of a society in which children are cherished likely go far beyond the elimination of malnutrition and direct mistreatment. He argues that the effects of a stable family structure and maternal affection produce healthier, taller, more disease-resistant and more intelligent children. Later in this book, the abundant evidence of a link between psychological status and life expectancy will be explored. It seems self-evident that such a link proves critical in infancy and early childhood.

It is now time to consider the case of the "Dog That Didn't Bark." In one of the most famous adventures of Sherlock Holmes, the critical clue was not some tiny piece of evidence, shrewdly observed and analyzed. It was an expected event that failed to occur—the dog that didn't bark.

Even though our analysis has downplayed the direct role of public health, immunization and medical intervention, the focus on direct evidence may underestimate the magnitude of their contribution. What manner of devastating epidemics might have been prevented? What outbreaks of disease were contained?

The role of nuclear weapons provides another analogy. On direct evidence, it might be argued that nuclear devices have been used only twice, and never decided the outcome of any war, large or small. However, it is much more accurate to say that nuclear weapons have influenced the nature of every conflict since their discovery by transforming the fundamental terms in which destruction and war are considered.

For example, consider a comparable case from the world of microscopic life-forms. After an absence of almost two centuries, the bubonic plague appeared in Asia beginning in 1894. After causing tens of thousands of deaths in China and India, it was contained, in part through controlling the rat that carried the infected fleas. However, the plague also died out in Asian populations where it was not well controlled. So it cannot be said for certain that intentional countermeasures prevented another worldwide epidemic. But it can be argued confidently that once the roles of fleas and rats were understood, the advanced nations had the tools to protect themselves from this particular devastation. As the populations in the advanced nations got healthier, conditions for transmission became more difficult, and health status was monitored with greater care, the opportunities for a new epidemic were reduced, although certainly not eliminated. Therefore, the unsung achievements of medical care and public health may well be the bugs that didn't bite.

With the last important piece of the puzzle now in place, it becomes possible to observe the broad picture of the great gain in human longevity. The whole is much greater than the sum of the parts because each of the parts interacts. The benefits of a stable and loving family on child mortality could not be achieved in a world still decimated by the bubonic plague. While it may be that nutrition was not the key factor, it is equally hard to imagine a public works program to clean up water and food in a community where people were starving wholesale. The interventions of medical care are infinitely more effective in a context where the patient population is fundamentally healthy and well-fed. Consider what Thucydides tells us in the oldest detailed account of an epidemic. He reports that the worst may not have been the disease itself, which struck down thousands. People shunned the gods and started living for the moment. Family responsibilities were ignored and civic order declined. It likely works both ways: the burden of disease falls heavily on social organization and civic order; advances in these also improve underlying health status.

A whole that is greater than the sum of the interacting parts suggests it might be possible to change any single factor without much affecting overall longevity. This helps explain why, as noted earlier in the book, similar life expectancies were observed over a wide range of medical systems, ranging from the very basic to the elaborate and extraordinarily expensive. If executed prudently, it is likely that a large cutback in spending for medical care could be achieved without much affecting life expectancy. In World War II the British discovered to their surprise that the nutritional cutbacks required by wartime rationing did not increase mortality rates—and may have been why death rates fell.

Sometimes there are two routes to the same objective. For example, one study of infant mortality concluded that it could be reduced by either of two strategies: a program of counseling, nutrition and prenatal care for unmarried teenage mothers to reduce the incidence of premature, underweight babies; or creation of more specialized prenatal intensive care units in hospitals so that more premature babies survived. This particular author concluded that in this instance the intensive medical technology solution would be cheaper than the social program, but, in general, medical solutions have proved quite expensive.

Observe all the pieces of the puzzle at work in the story of a young and idealistic New York physician named Michael Alderman. With a Harvard education and an M.D. from Yale, Alderman was looking for a chance to make a difference. The year was 1972. He soon found himself in a remote mountain community in Jamaica, heading a project to reduce an astronomical infant mortality rate. With his medical training and the help of Cornell University medical students, he was going to save babies with the miracle of modern medical care.

But for many weeks Alderman was both mystified and frustrated. Babies would be brought to him suffering from nothing more than mild diarrhea and maybe a rash—hardly a medical emergency. But soon he learned the babies had died. He was having little impact.

Then he began to circulate around the mountain homes, and instead of trying to cure the sick babies, he started weighing all of them. Quickly he learned that the unexpected deaths were occurring among those that were badly underweight. And when he focused on those who were underweight, he found they had been weaned early and weren't getting enough protein in their diet. Alderman ultimately succeeded in reducing the infant mortality rate by weighing babies and handing out free protein supplements for the undernourished, underweight infants.

So why did more babies survive and life expectancy increase in the mountains of Jamaica? Official statistics would show a decline in deaths from diarrheal diseases. Unmistakably, nutrition was improved in the most fragile of human populations. Cornell University Medical School might see proof that to save lives in a primitive area, the answer was to send them a smart doctor. A public health official would say the solution lay in the domain of epidemiology—and the careful measurement of the occurrence of illness. Sagan might say it was better care for vulnerable infants.

To unravel the separate threads of the cloth is to risk losing sight of the pattern. These factors are woven inextricably together, each interacting with the others, to produce the longest human lifespans the world has ever known. One should, however, rejoice in this great accomplishment with caution. The next chapters will explore the important and neglected question of whether the longevity gains wrested from the teeming world of microscopic life might be rapidly reversed.

CHAPTER FIVE

GOD DOES PLAY DICE

On a balmy morning in late January 1991, seven men and two women gathered in a conference room near Washington, D.C., to make a decision that would affect thousands of lives. The principals with seats at the front table were all senior physicians with long experience in the sobering business of life and death judgments. Unlike military generals, who may dispatch entire armies to victory or defeat, doctors usually make their decisions on a case-by-case basis. This day, however, would be different. The morning's agenda would affect 30 million Americans and might mark the difference between life and death for thousands of persons.

The group is officially known as the Vaccines and Related Biological Products Advisory Committee, and its members are primarily immunologists and pediatricians from medical schools. It assists the federal Food and Drug Administration. The task today was to recommend the ingredients of a vaccine that would be given to more Americans over the next year than any other such product. The target was a disease that in an average year kills 10,000 persons in the United States. In a bad year—which occurs every decade or two—it could claim 100,000 lives. And in a very bad year—and there have been just two this century—the death toll might reach 1 million. The group gathered at FDA headquarters would recommend a vaccine they hoped would help counter the inevitable upcoming attack from the single most successful predator of mankind: the influenza virus.

The flu seems such a ubiquitous annoyance that it is easy to overlook the fact that it is the only force at large today that has repeatedly shortened the overall human life expectancy in the United States in this century. In the past forty years alone, influenza has reduced life expectancy in the United States six times: in 1957, 1960, 1963, 1968, 1980 and 1988. In at least three of these flu epidemics, there was a serious mismatch between the disease and the contents or quantity of the vaccine.

Here is a virus that kills by the thousand, infects by the million, closes schools, decimates conferences and paralyzes hospitals. The impossible choices it may present a nation without warning may have cost a President of the United States—Gerald Ford—his office. In six months' time it sweeps across the steppes of central Asia, cuts a swath through the billions in China, rolls through the Mediterranean world and into Europe. It may leap the ocean to enter the Western Hemisphere from either coast. The threat in the United States usually ends with spring, but the virus then moves to the Southern Hemisphere where winter approaches.

We are not without defenses. Although the virus was not isolated until 1933, influenza is perhaps the most carefully studied, well-characterized and thoroughly understood human virus. Every character of the genetic instructions written into the RNA of the influenza virus has been decoded. For the most important entries in the virus's genetic code book, virologists at the Centers for Disease Control will notice if a single letter has changed. This is like being so familiar with a community's telephone book that a new number for a single customer is immediately noticed. The characteristics of the circulating viruses are monitored by a worldwide surveillance network joined by 76 nations and coordinated by the United Nations World Health Organization. A flu vaccine has been available since 1943. Under most circumstances, the transmission of a flu virus particle can be prevented by a simple paper face mask.

For all this, influenza rages through the human population at will, almost entirely untamed. On three occasions since 1950 the United States has contemplated heroic countermeasures to an anticipated onslaught of major proportions. All three efforts were failures. Each year a modest immunization program is promoted to reduce the death toll among the elderly and those with respiratory disease. It has little effect. A more virulent flu strain is almost certain to appear, although it is impossible to know whether this might occur in 6 months or 60 years. There is no plan to combat this predictable threat. This is not simply an obvious failure of policy or foresight by the nation's influenza warriors. At least in part, the problem is embedded in the molecular design of a virus whose threat to human beings changes at random.

Such random changes seem alien to the human desires to plan and predict, to live in an orderly world. When a frustrated Albert Einstein wrote that "God does not play dice with the universe," he was resisting the inherent unpredictability embodied in quantum mechanics. However, the problems raised by the uncertainty principle look tame next to the wide-open craps game that the flu virus plays continually with the genetic code in which its very existence is written. Not only is God playing dice, He has offered up thousands and possibly millions of human lives as the table stakes. And when mankind steps up to the craps table to play for the next year's flu vaccine, the very best the most knowledgeable experts in the world can hope for is a lucky guess. In the FDA conference room near Washington, that was the morning's task.

While the next flu season would not begin for at least nine months, the committee members soon learned that, already, time was of the essence. The session was chaired by Roland Levandowski, a physician in the FDA branch that licenses vaccines.

"There are some realities of production of vaccine that I would like to review very briefly," said Levandowski. "The manufacturers have to begin to decide how many doses of vaccine they will be able to manufacture," he said. Flu vaccine is manufactured from flu virus that is grown in chicken embryos inside eggs, and then inactivated. He noted, "That includes determining what the size of their flock should be so they get an adequate number of eggs. That is already going on." Levandowski didn't say this, but the current realities of flu vaccine production meant the committee would have to guess what strains might circulate next year before much data were available for the current year. This meant, for example, that if an unexpected new strain emerged over the summer in the Southern Hemisphere, it would be difficult if not impossible to react.

The first step, however, was to examine the current flu season, where something unusual had already occurred. Louisa Chapman, of the CDC epidemiology branch, reported the latest findings from the CDC's four nationwide and one worldwide flu surveillance systems. The influenza virus is classified into three types, labeled A, B, and C. The influenza A virus is the most feared and dominant type, and infects humans, seals, pigs, birds, ferrets, whales, mink and cattle. Occasionally a near relative, influenza B, causes an epidemic in humans, but has never been seen in animals. Much less is known about influenza C, and few steps are taken to combat it. Needless to say, immunity to influenza A provides little or no protection against influenza B. Chapman tells the committee that for the first time in a decade, the influenza B virus appears to be the predominant type in circulation, a major change from the previous year when a serious epidemic was almost entirely due to influenza A.

In the weeks before Christmas, influenza B swept through areas of the Northeast, where it closed down entire schools, often infecting 30 percent of the children. Since this type B had not circulated since 1980, virtually no young children had immunity to the virus. However unpleasant and worrying an experience it may have provided to millions of parents of infected children, this influenza B strain was proving to be mild. Because it is difficult and expensive to isolate a virus, the CDC uses indirect methods to measure the lethality of the strain. Each week it monitors all deaths from pneumonia and influenza in 127 cities. If such deaths exceed an expected number during the flu season, it is assumed that influenza is responsible for the excess mortality. At this point early in the flu season, there is yet no indication of excess deaths from the flu, Chapman tells the committee. Influenza A has been occasionally reported, but mostly it is a milder type B. "We are very fortunate," she says.

There was another reason to conclude that the nation had indeed been fortunate with the B virus. A vaccine may provide protection from one strain of the type B virus, but have little or no effect on another. The previous year, two major strains of the B virus had been detected, B/Yamagata and B/Victoria, each named after the city where it was first detected and classified. The committee decided to bet on B/Yamagata, which was included in the vaccine. In England it turned out that B/Victoria accounted for half the cases, and B/Yamagata the other half. However, in the United States, the early returns showed that the B virus was basically similar to the B/Yamagata strain in the vaccine, not a perfect match, but well within the bounds of the immunologically useful. This time the committee had put its money on the right number and won.

Luck had not held, however, with an A virus vaccine component.

They had to make a choice between two different strains from China, denoted A/Shanghai and A/Beijing. The committee had recommended Shanghai, which was similar to the strain then circulating in the United States. A year later, viruses now being isolated in the United States unfortunately looked more like A/Beijing.

This meant the vaccine provided much less effective protection. "The percentage of people who developed what would be considered protective levels was only about half of what was seen with A/Shanghai/16/89 strain," the FDA's Levandowski told the committee.

If few cases of this strain of influenza A appeared in the United States, and the B type predominated, the partial vaccine mismatch might turn out to be of little importance. If an A/Beijing virus swept through with the force of the preceding year, thousands of elderly persons might die despite their flu vaccination. The 1990 vaccine was trivalent, providing protection against three strains of flu, one type B, and two type A. The third component, targeted against another type A strain, needed no changes.

As the advisory meeting progressed, it became increasingly evident that the dominant voice in the room was not a committee member or FDA official. It was coming from a slender, soft-spoken Englishman named Alan Kendal. As chief of the influenza branch of the federal Centers for Disease Control, Kendal was the nation's top flu warrior. A microbiologist by training, Kendal had received his doctorate for a study of one of the protein spikes that protrudes from the flu virus capsule. His style, however, was not of the domineering commander, but of a quiet committee-oriented consensus manager.

Kendal had a delicate problem to raise with the committee, a development that no one wanted to see blazing across the newspaper headlines. From Denver, Colorado, the CDC had received reports of two cases of a rare form of rapidly developing paralysis called Guillain-Barré syndrome. A syndrome is the most mysterious of all human disorders. It describes a related group of symptoms often occurring together. But no one knows what causes it: A virus? Bacterial invader? A genetic defect waiting some triggering event? With Guillain-Barré the most educated guesses focus on a disorder of the immune system that causes the body to attack its own nerve cells. In both the public and medical mind, however, the immediate and obvious connection is with flu shots. In

1976 a nationwide mass immunization program ground entirely to a halt amidst reports of an association with Guillain-Barré. Since then, the CDC had not observed the association again, although Kendal said they had stopped monitoring the situation after observing nothing for the next two years.

Kendal told the committee that they had now found two cases of Guillain-Barré in Denver. They occurred in two elderly patients in the same intensive care unit of one hospital. Both patients had recently gotten flu vaccinations from the same health maintenance organization. Kendal expressed concern that if the CDC went looking for Guillain-Barré cases associated with flu shots they would immediately find them, in a kind of self-fulfilling prophecy—because some cases will occur anyway, and millions of flu shots were being given.

"There is a strong potential for bias in reporting. That is, when there is an investigation conducted looking for GBS [Guillain-Barré syndrome], there is likely to be an automatic response to try to identify cases where the vaccine is the cause or is temporally associated."

But Kendal was also plainly worried about the publicity. "There is no evidence of a clear problem here that would warrant any statements being made that would be unduly alarming and potentially damage influenza vaccination unnecessarily," he said.

The CDC did not advertise this, but it was not greatly successful in persuading the medical community and the elderly to participate in the immunization program. By most estimates, only about 20 percent got annual shots and any bad publicity might dramatically reduce this figure. CDC also did not publicize the fact that the vaccine was not especially effective in the elderly. In CDC's largest study, focusing on seven Michigan nursing homes, vaccine reduced the incidence of flu infections from 33 percent to 21 percent of the residents. Its effect on mortality was more impressive: 1.1 percent of those vaccinated died, compared with 4.4 percent of the unvaccinated.

The Guillain-Barré cases were a public health, public relations and scientific dilemma wrapped into one horrifying package. Here was a rare condition, a group of related symptoms not invariably diagnosed and not routinely reported. Even in the documented instances where it was associated with the 1976 swine flu vaccine, there was only 1 case for every 100,000 persons vaccinated.

If they made a major announcement, getting the publicity needed to find the rare cases, they might sink the flu immunization program. On the other hand, if they moved too quietly they might, by mistake, dismiss the Denver cases as a fluke because they never found out about other incidents. What if, for example, Guillain-Barré was triggered by a contaminant in the vaccines, something present in 1976 that was now getting back into the United States supplies?

The CDC solution, Kendal told the committee, was to launch a quiet investigation, piggybacking on an existing study of the cost effectiveness of the flu vaccine being conducted in 10 states.

In a world where medical treatment is too often sold to the public as all benefits and no risks, it is easy to see why CDC wanted to keep quiet about a potential risk not yet confirmed. And finally, Kendal was introducing a serious bias in the opposite direction. The public has a genuine reason to worry about the bias, conscious or unconscious, that might occur in a secret investigation of an important complication to flu vaccination conducted by the same agency that is already promoting it to the public as safe and effective. It would take time to complete a proper study, Kendal told the committee.

When it came to recommending a 1991 vaccine, the committee approved Kendal's proposals with little debate and no modification. The vaccine would include protection against two type A strains and one type B strain. If they were lucky, one of these three strains—or a close relative—would actually circulate the next fall. For the 1991–1992 flu season, the bets were down. Now the dice would roll.

That meeting at the FDA gives a glimpse of the resources that science and medicine can deploy to combat flu. It is equally revealing to examine what occurred when the full menace of the influenza virus was brought to bear on human civilization.

The Army soldier was admitted to the base hospital at Fort Devens, Massachusetts, with a soaring fever and an unproductive cough. To the young attending physician, this was not a typical case of pneumonia, which often runs a course of 10 days or more. This patient was literally getting worse by the minute. Darkened patches began to appear on the cheekbones, a condition called cyanosis that results from insufficient oxygen in the blood. Then the darkened areas appeared around the ears and spread across the whole face. It got worse and worse until, in the words of one attending physician: "It was simply a struggle for air until he suffocated. It was horrible."

More such patients arrived at the Fort Devens hospital. The physician remarked: "One can stand it to see one, two or twenty men die, but to see the poor devils dropping out like flies sort of gets on your nerves. We have been averaging a hundred deaths per day."

The date was September 1918. A disease dubbed "the Spanish flu" had arrived in the United States, and the worst epidemic in United States history had begun. The year had already been among the most tumultuous in history. World War I raged in full force. In just six months' time, the United States had poured more than one million troops into Europe, probably the largest mass movement of humans in history. There, in the muddy trenches of France, they rubbed shoulders with Europeans, Indians, Africans, Australians and Egyptians. It was the perfect target of opportunity for a virus. Earlier, in the spring, the last massive German offensive bogged down, and later the general in command would blame influenza for decimating the divisions on the critical left wing of the attack. Flu swept through battalions, laid up the crews of entire ships and immobilized training bases. But up until September this was no killer. It was just another flu epidemic, a briefly debilitating fever and period of weakness, making the most of a world in which traditional patterns had been disrupted as millions were gathered from around the world for the slaughter on the fields of France.

Then something happened. Nobody knows for sure what. Alfred W. Crosby, Jr., in a widely quoted history of the pandemic, cites a specific event in Africa. If it did not mark the actual beginning of the pandemic, it must have been an incident something like this. On August 15, 1918, His Majesty's Ship *Mantua* put in to harbor in Sierra Leone on the west coast of Africa. The ship needed to replenish its coal bunkers. When it docked, at least 200 sailors were down with the flu, apparently picked up in the previous port of call in Europe. There is no evidence any of the flu cases were unusually serious. Native black laborers loaded the ship with coal, and it departed without incident. A week later, port physicians noted some cases that resembled flu. Two weeks after the ship had first arrived, 500 of the 600 laborers who had loaded the ship were ill. It was later estimated that two-thirds of the population of Sierra Leone caught the flu. In the port city alone, then called Freetown, more than 1,000 died. Ships calling at Sierra Leone soon began to report large numbers of crew deaths in the days after their port visit. Thirty-eight died on the *Chepstow Castle,* and sixty-eight on the *Tahiti.* Had the flu virus undergone some lethal mutation as it ripped through an African population with little immunity? The twentieth-century world was about to experience the global devastation of disease that spread with a speed and lethality never seen before in history.

It reached the city limits of Philadelphia, Pennsylvania, on September 28, the date when 200,000 citizens packed the streets for a parade to promote war bonds. Here was a perfect location for the flu to strike. It was ringed with military installations: Philadelphia Navy Yard right in town, Fort Meade nearby in Maryland, and in neighboring New Jersey, Fort Dix. In the week ending October 5, a total of 706 persons died of flu. But the next week the death toll tripled; in seven days' more time, it doubled again. The peak occurred in Philadelphia during the week of October 19, 1918, when 4,597 persons died. So many people died so quickly there were no coffins available, and too few gravediggers and undertakers. As the morgues overflowed, bodies were stacked up in huge cold-storage warehouses until someone could attend to them. Schools, churches, theaters and saloons were closed. There were so many abandoned children with sick or dead parents that civic authorities simply asked neighbors to take them in. Then, like a wave that has crested, the deaths began to decline nearly as rapidly as they had risen. In the week ending November 30, just 93 died of influenza or pneumonia.

The influenza, however, moved on. It struck hard in New York, Chicago and San Francisco, but mostly bypassed Cleveland and Indianapolis. The toll continued in other cities as the flu season continued into the opening months of 1919. It reappeared again, in somewhat more benign form, in 1920, and then disappeared forever, reverting back to the familiar, vastly less lethal virus. In the United States it killed about 550,000 persons overall out of a population of 125 million. The worldwide toll is conventionally but crudely estimated at 20 million. However, some believe the real toll might have been double that.

The reasons for the unusual lethality of the 1918 flu virus are uncertain, and debated to this day. Some series of autopsies of flu victims showed a pattern of bacterial infection that suggested flu increased vulnerability to secondary pneumonia or strep infection. This reassuring school of thought holds a recurrence is impossible in the modern antibiotic era. Most analysts concede some of the excess mortality came from this source. But did this account for all of it? Another theory backs a mysterious "cofactor"—another organism that just happened to circulate simultaneously but might not have been lethal unless teamed with the flu virus. The debate about 1918 can't be settled with the evidence that survives. "Probably the virus was unusually virulent," concluded Mt. Sinai Medical School's Edwin Kilbourne, a prominent flu researcher. What is certain is that flu viruses now in circulation have the genetic potential to become substantially more virulent. Furthermore, later studies of antibodies in blood samples allowed a tentative identification of the 1918 strain. It was an influenza A virus quite similar to a strain still circulating among pigs. The popular nickname is the swine flu.

The influenza virus shares with humans a claim on being among the most successful life-forms the world has ever known. But it would be hard to conceive of anything built of the same common materials of life that achieved this goal by a more drastically different strategy. To examine an influenza A particle is to see the rudiments of life stripped down to such stark essentials that the result is not, strictly speaking, even alive at all. The chief wonder here is how something so simple could make so much trouble.

Seen from the outside in an electron microscope photograph, the influenza virus particle is spherical in shape, studded with small protruding spikes. A majority of the spikes are shaped like a round-headed nail that is called the HA or hemagglutinin protein. In the lungs, the rounded heads of the HA spikes latch onto receptors in the cell membrane like the interlocking teeth of a zipper. Once tightly attached, the virus is absorbed into the cell. Once inside, the virus takes command of the cell's machinery to produce thousands of component parts of new viral particles, ultimately wrecking the cell beyond repair. As the viral particles depart the ruined cell, they get an assist from the other, smaller class of spikes studding the spherical exterior: the NA, or neuraminidase, spikes help prevent the particles from getting stuck to the fatty cell membrane.

One of the human body's chief defenses against influenza is anti-bodies, the Y-shaped molecules that attach to very specific sites on the surface of a virus, in lock-and-key fashion. In this part of the immune defense, the body tests the viral particle for distinctive locks on its surface, and then manufactures a large quantity of keys. When antibodies are attached to the protruding HA spikes of the viral particle, it cannot latch onto a living cell and enter it.

Faced with human immune systems that can quickly manufacture keys, the virus counters with an exceptional capacity to change the lock through mutation. In human cells, the genetic code is carefully safe-guarded against mutation by being wound into two-stranded helixes of DNA. Only when a segment of code is needed to manufacture a particu-lar protein is it translated into the more fragile single strands of RNA. But the influenza virus consists only of strands of the less stable RNA. This allows it to mutate 100,000 to 1 million times more rapidly than the DNA in human cells. Most of the mutations, of course, are worth-less. But nature tries everything, at random, and sooner or later, one of the mutations changes the shape of the locations where antibodies at-tach. A change in a single molecule—if it is exactly the right one—will defeat the antibody immune response. This process is called genetic drift, and it is one reason that one year's flu vaccine may not be effective against the next year's virus. Fortunately, there are several sites on a flu virus where different antibodies attach. The usual effect of genetic drift is a slow and continual reduction in the effectiveness of the immune response.

Embedded in the design of the flu virus particle is an even more dramatic capacity for transformation. The genetic code of a flu virus particle is packaged into eight tiny protein capsules. In about every one or two billionth infected individual, a special event may occur. The particles from two entirely different viral strains enter the same cell. Both particles set the machinery of the cell to work, manufacturing the com-ponents of a virus. Simple mathematics tells us that, with two copies of eight different RNA capsules, in a stroke we have 256 possible viruses. This process is something like creating a new house pet combining the mouth of a dog, the tail of a cat and the wings of a bird. This is called genetic shift, and it means that, in terms of immune response, an entirely new virus can emerge in a single master stroke.

Genetic shift, therefore, has produced dramatic flu outbreaks that are global in scope. At today's population totals, a newly shifted virus might produce one billion cases of influenza in the first 24 months. Even with a fairly mild strain of influenza, that amounts to a cost of 1 million lives. In the United States alone the losses might reach 100,000. Such a global event is described as a pandemic, to distinguish it from more localized outbreaks, which are called epidemics. The most recent global pandemics following genetic shift occurred in 1957 and 1968, and in both years the impact was large enough to reduce life expectancy in the United States.

Within the coded RNA of influenza lies another important possibility. Either through the small changes of genetic drift, or new combinations of entire strands of RNA, influenza can suddenly gain or lose virulence. Any change that makes a virus more effective in attaching to, entering, replicating in or exiting a human cell makes it more virulent. It means more viral particles to spread, and more human cells destroyed. An increase in virulence might mean a flu that left its victim bedridden for a week instead of 24 hours. It might also turn flu into a much more lethal killer. This possibility provided the model for Stephen King's best-selling fictional account of the end of the civilized world, *The Stand,* and Michael Crichton's story of its near demise, *The Andromeda Strain.*

These fictional scenarios lie uncomfortably close to scientific fact. There is a specific, known location in the genetic code of influenza A which, if altered ever so slightly, would dramatically increase its virulence. This change in genetic code could be accomplished, with known techniques, in many of the microbiology laboratories that routinely use and modify viruses for a wide variety of purposes.

The CDC's Kendal concedes such a possibility exists. "It is theoretically possible," he said. "Based on published research techniques it is clearly possible to do it. But there's no guarantee that the end product would survive. Certainly none of us are going to do the experiment to reconstruct a human influenza virus with such a sequence change."

At the same time, however, Kendal describes doomsday scenarios as "farfetched." A doomsday virus would have to be more virulent, be biologically viable, and evade the existing immune defenses. Nobody today, he says, knows how to do all three simultaneously.

It was, however, a fear of the consequences of genetic shift and increase in virulence that set the stage for the first systematic effort to combat a flu pandemic. By the year 1957 medical science could detect, isolate and identify many viruses. A flu vaccine had been manufactured routinely for more than a decade. And the disease was already the target of coordinated global vigilance, fueled by the still-vivid memories of 1918.

In April of 1957 word came from Hong Kong that the flu was sweeping through the crowded city with unusual force. Then it leaped to Shanghai and Manila and spread into the jungles of southeast Asia. It aroused no immediate concern until virologists in London, Melbourne and Washington simultaneously discovered it was being caused by a new influenza A subtype created by genetic shift. This subtype had probably not circulated through the world since 1899, so it would encounter a world population largely without acquired immune defenses. What made this development of special interest to the world's epidemiologists was that this event had been specifically and explicitly predicted. Exactly 11 years after the last major new subtype had appeared in 1946, genetic shift had occurred again. In roughly one-year's time it was expected to conquer the world, arriving in the United States in force in the next flu season.

In the Southern Hemisphere where winter was approaching, nature was left to take its course. Since the United States had more resources and more lead time, the scientific and medical community decided to fight back. As committees of experts contemplated the nation's response, a whole series of agonizing problems arose. Could enough vaccine be produced to immunize a whole nation? Probably not, but the manufacturers could make at least 50 million doses. But the scientific community would have to hope that the new influenza A subtype was the only strain that would circulate. That was so the industry could manufacture three times as many doses of a monovalent, or one-part, vaccine as it could the normal trivalent product. Who should be protected first? The elderly, the most likely to die of the flu? Or children, who were most likely to be infected and least likely to resist it? What about essential personnel? Most of these decisions were left to state and local health organizations. The manufacturers, meanwhile, moved to maximum production.

The new flu strain first surfaced in the United States in April. The pharmaceutical industry got a sample on May 12, 1957. It immediately began to experiment to see how much vaccine it could produce. Initial results were terrible, yielding only about one weak dose per embryonic egg. By the end of July, the pharmaceutical industry had mostly beaten the technical problems. Production began to grow exponentially. By the middle of October the industry was producing nearly 7 million vaccine doses every week. Forecasts of total production were raised practically every week. It might be possible to manufacture 85 million doses of vaccine by the end of February.

None of this vast effort had a useful effect. Given the size and scale of the problem, the industry reacted quickly. But the flu virus arrived too soon. On June 2 it struck at the Navy base in Newport, Rhode Island. Three weeks later it was detected among teenage girls at a conference near Sacramento, California. Any doubt it would take hold in the United States was largely eliminated when it struck 250 of 1,800 youths who had gathered from 43 states for a Boy Scout Jamboree in Grinnell, Iowa. The epidemic did not peak until the middle of October 1957. At that time, vaccine was just beginning to arrive in millions of doses, but the initial supplies were weak and of limited effectiveness. In many areas, much of the public was simply not interested in vaccination. The United States scientific and medical establishment had run a race with a flu strain whose appearance had been long predicted, and it had lost completely. The resulting cost in lives totaled 85,000.

Eleven years later, in 1968, it would happen again. A new subtype suddenly appeared in Hong Kong and swept the globe. The results of the U.S. response, in the words of Edwin Kilbourne, were "insignificant." The excess mortality: 33,000 lives. Another eight years later, in 1976, Kilbourne warned that the nation was no better prepared this time, when once again, a global pandemic would occur. The events that actually took place would surprise even the veteran flu scientist Kilbourne.

.   .   .

In late January 1976, the Army hospital at Fort Dix, New Jersey, was filling up with new recruits running a high fever and a respiratory infection. In basic training it is commonplace for 20 percent of every unit to contract some kind of minor respiratory disorder. One of the constant challenges for the cadre is separating those who are really sick from those who are just sick of the Army. There are large numbers of both. But even to the seasoned medical staff of Fort Dix, it was clear something unusual was going on, an exceptional number of cases of acute respiratory disease. There were 35 hospitalized the first week, then 53. By the fourth week there were 173.

Colonel Joseph D. Bartley, the post's chief of preventative medicine, believed he had identified the cause: adenovirus 21. That was what the report from the Army's Walter Reed Laboratory said, based on samples taken the first week in the new year. This family of 33 viruses accounts for many a case of fever, cough and swollen adenoids in children. It is not often seen elsewhere except in military recruits. As a courtesy, however, the county health department would be notified. With 5,000 dependents on post, rare was the outbreak that couldn't leap from the base into the civilian community, and vice versa. The date was January 27, 1976.

The very next day Bartley was on the phone to the New Jersey Department of Public Health. Dr. Martin Goldfield, the assistant commissioner and chief epidemiologist, wanted to know what was going on. Bartley filled him in on the suspected adenovirus epidemic. Goldfield, however, had a different theory. He thought an outbreak that explosive could only be influenza. In fact, Goldfield would bet money on it. Thus it happened that Colonel Bartley sent over eight containers of fluid with which eight different ailing recruits had gargled. The next day, Friday, Bartley sent over eleven more samples.

In Goldfield's laboratory the samples were inoculated into 10-day-old embryonic chicks and incubated over the weekend. On Monday the laboratory staff set to work to isolate any virus that had been growing in the embryos. They found influenza virus in six of the samples. In four, the staff immediately identified A/Victoria, a familiar strain that was already forcing area schools to close and creating absentee problems for large businesses.

But two samples were a complete mystery. There was evidence that the samples were a flu virus of some kind. But they were not among the influenza strains known to be circulating through the world. The New Jersey virology laboratory was part of the World Health Organization's global network and had serum samples at hand for the circulating strains. Goldfield was soon on the telephone to the Centers for Disease Control in Atlanta. He talked to Walter Dowdle, who was then chief of the influenza branch. This was probably nothing, he told Dowdle, but he was going to send him some samples of an influenza virus that they couldn't identify in New Jersey. It appeared to be a radically new strain of influenza. He would put them on the plane that very night.

The same day Goldstein also called back the medical staff at Fort Dix. Indeed they did have a flu epidemic at the post, even though every recruit was vaccinated on the day of arrival, and the cadre every October. The post medics were not exactly surprised. They had observed that an unusual number of those hospitalized had recently arrived on post. It takes two weeks to build immunity after vaccination. The virus doesn't always wait that long. Then Goldstein said something that put in motion a chain of events that would affect the whole nation. Because they had isolated a still-unidentified flu virus, he suggested that if any recruit died they should be sure to get a throat swab to send over for analysis.

Two days later Private David Lewis, 19 years old, had spent the day in the barracks with a fever and cough. Fearing he might not graduate on schedule if he missed any more training, he joined his company in a grueling five-mile night march. Shortly thereafter he died.

By the end of the week the New Jersey Health Department laboratory had finished work on all the samples from Fort Dix. Six were unmistakably specimens of A/Victoria then circulating through New Jersey. There were also five cases of the mystery flu strain. One of them came from David Lewis, deceased.

Another week elapsed before the CDC laboratory identified the mystery strain of influenza. It was a type A strain found in pigs. Occasionally it was isolated from humans who proved to have directly contracted it from pigs. It produced a mild illness. Since there were no pigs at Fort Dix, it was virtually certain that this virus strain was now being transmitted from person to person. It had one more characteristic that would make it famous around the world. No one can determine what strain of influenza virus circulated in 1918. It was known, however, that many people who had been alive in 1918 or the early 1920s had antibodies to this swine flu strain. So it must have circulated widely among humans in that period, although the flu strains of the 1920s were not unusually virulent. Now five soldiers had gotten the swine flu in 1976, and one was dead. That very evening, Dowdle called the director of the CDC, David J. Sencer, to tell him it appeared the swine flu was on the loose once again.

On the government organization chart, the Centers for Disease Control looks like just another agency buried in the belly of the behemoth currently named the Department of Health and Human Services. Nothing could be more misleading. In the area of infectious disease, the Centers for Disease Control is an elite organization that is renowned in scientific circles the world over. To a young physician, a two-year appointment to the Epidemiological Intelligence Service, or EIS, has the same prestige and glamour that lawyers find in the chance to clerk for a Supreme Court justice. The CDC keeps many of the best and brightest veterans of the EIS. And from that group came the senior staff and director. And among the top echelons of CDC are some of the most savvy and experienced civil servants the government has ever seen, equipped with not only scientific and medical training, but years of experience in how to move the cranky, complex machinery of the United States government. And like so many among the scientific and medical elite, they do not lack confidence.

Into the domain of David J. Sencer, director of the CDC, came the treacherous problem of five cases of the swine flu detected at Fort Dix, New Jersey. He was a dominating figure at CDC, with an influence so pervasive that he once bragged he personally reviewed every promotion down to the level of janitor. There were only a few things that Sencer could know for certain. If a vaccine protecting against swine flu was going to be available for the flu season beginning next October, a decision would have to be made quickly. The industry was already churning out doses to immunize against the A/Victoria strain now circulating. So any decision by necessity would have to be made before knowing how lethal the swine flu might be, and whether in fact it would create a worldwide pandemic, or any further cases at all. This is the inevitable dilemma forced by a virus that can change and spread rapidly, pitted against a system that reacts quite slowly.

A great deal is known about what happened next. Two famous Harvard professors, Richard E. Neustadt and Harvey V. Fineberg, were later provided with complete access to the participants and confidential government records. The resulting book, *The Swine Flu Affair,* is a classic analysis of the perils of scientific decision-making at high levels of government, and was an important source for this account.

After meeting with senior scientists in the government and medical community, Sencer decided to advocate flu shots for everyone, a full-blown, nationwide immunization program. He soon fired off a memorandum, a political silver bullet so skillfully aimed that, within two days, the issue had landed on the desk of the president of the United States, Gerald Ford. The date was March 15, 1976.

Coming from the government's senior expert on infectious disease, the third paragraph of Sencer's memorandum is probably all any president needed to see: "The virus is antigenically related to the influenza virus that has been implicated in the cause of the 1918–1919 pandemic which killed 450,000 people—more than 400 of every 100,000 Americans."

When accompanied by the statement that a decision had to be made now if vaccine were to be available, it was, as Neustadt and Fineberg put it, the equivalent of holding a gun to the head of the president of the United States. At this point, how could he respond, "Gosh, let's not do anything." Not only was this dire statement in a confidential government memorandum, Sencer had made a similar comparison in an earlier press conference in response to a question.

While President Ford couldn't get off the shaky limb onto which he had been forced, he could and did get plenty of company. What happened next is an important but dismal chapter in the history of rational policy for infectious disease.

On March 24, 1976, Ford walked into the cabinet room at the White House. Arrayed around the polished walnut table were some of the most famous names in infectious disease and public health. Sencer and Kilbourne were there. So were the two great polio vaccine scientists, Jonas Salk and Albert Sabin.

It was almost as if Ford smelled trouble coming. He asked for a show of hands by those who supported a massive national immunization program. Around the table, everyone raised a hand. Maybe some of those present had some private doubts, Ford said. So he halted the meeting and went to the Oval Office next door. Anyone who wanted to whisper privately in his ear could do so. No one came.

To be fair to the participants, it should be noted the group was hastily assembled; some of those invited were even coached by CDC officials on what they should say. However, if they in fact had doubts, it was their responsibility to express them. Much, much more was to go wrong as the swine flu immunization campaign moved forward. But already several disastrous mistakes had been made.

To have portrayed the swine flu as "antigenically related" to the 1918 strain was technically correct, but entirely misleading. Sencer and CDC's choice of such an inaccurate and inflammatory comparison would wreck any possibility of a rational consideration of the alternatives.

Certain facts were known before the immunization program was officially launched. The lethality of the 1918 flu strain had nothing to do with its antigenic character. For other reasons it was unusually virulent. Later "antigenically related" strains were not particularly virulent and circulated through humans for many years. Any strain, new or old, can suddenly change in virulence at any time, through either gradual genetic drift or the more dramatic reconfiguration of the virus that occurs in genetic shift.

To seasoned physicians, the death of a single recruit under unusual circumstances was not an indication of virulence. It was common knowledge among military medics that vigorous exercise could turn a mild, ordinary flu infection into a deadly affliction. Also, even ordinary flu strains often proved deadly. For example, in the New Jersey area in the same period, there were 12 deaths from ordinary A/Victoria, including the loss of an 11-day-old baby, a 31-year-old man with no preexisting disease and a 32-year-old woman who was previously in excellent health. Year in and year out, the case fatality rate of flu is 1 in 1,000.

By the time the medical luminaries assembled in the White House, there was already a growing body of evidence that the swine flu cases were probably a fluke. As soon as the swine flu virus was identified, investigators immediately launched an effort to monitor any spread of the disease. In over a month's time, not a single new case was identified. Nor could any be identified in the surrounding New Jersey communities, nor in any other state, either nearby or distant. In previous episodes with a strain to which little or no immunity was present, typical infection rates ranged from 20 to 30 percent of the exposed population. That could easily have totaled 4,000 cases at Fort Dix alone. But in the end, only 12 cases were found. In addition to the original 5, investigators located 7 other individuals who became ill about the same time, and proved to have the swine flu virus. Not even one additional case occurred after Private David Lewis died. Another several hundred recruits showed, by elevated antibodies, they had probably been exposed to the swine flu virus. But they did not become even slightly ill. This certainly did not make a case for an unusually virulent strain resembling the 1918 virus. But at least it is convincing enough to put to rest the otherwise serious possibility that the entire episode was triggered by a laboratory mixup. All these facts were known before a single swine flu shot was given, and before any doses were manufactured.

Still, the unknowns must have loomed large and frightening. Given the uncertainty embedded in the situation, it is hard to imagine another instance where the proverbial forbidden fruit from the tree of knowledge was sampled and provided such an immediately bitter taste: here was knowledge that did not make the future more manageable and certain; it made it less so. At a conference at the National Institutes of Health held a year later, it is almost possible to sense some of the participants wistfully recalling how close they came to never learning about the swine flu at all. If Private Lewis had just stayed in the barracks. If Goldfield just hadn't made his bet with Colonel Bartley about what really was circulating through Fort Dix. If the New Jersey Health Department labs had not been unusually skillful in handling the virus samples, the swine flu would have been missed entirely. These were scientists, the most devout of believers in the power of knowledge. One can almost sense some of the participants saying, maybe for the first time in their lives, this is something they would really rather not have known.

That's because once they knew about the swine flu, Sencer, Kilbourne and the others also had to consider the cost of doing nothing. What would the public say if a virulent flu strain swept the country the next fall and it emerged the CDC knew about it for eight months and did nothing? For many years the biomedical establishment had exaggerated its powers over the world of microscopic life-forms. The public outcry would be enormous. However, if the CDC could pull off a successful nationwide immunization program it might be a triumph for preventive medicine, even if this turned out to be quite a mild strain of flu. That's how it must have looked. What, in fact, happened was quite something else.

Credibility was the first casualty when President Ford publicly launched the national immunization effort. Given a medical or scientific question, the national news media are often remarkably meek and accepting when briefed by someone wrapped in proper credentials. But to witness the give-and-take of daily media coverage of the nation's top political leaders, including the president, is to enter a world where cynicism and skepticism are unbounded. Virtually the same day that Ford was identified with the swine flu immunization program, the airwaves and newspaper columns were filled with speculation that the swine flu was a dubious threat contrived for the political benefit of an embattled president.

Then the pharmaceutical companies threatened not to make the vaccine unless given legal immunity from anyone who was harmed rather than helped by their flu shot. It must be, they seemed to say, so dangerous to get an immunization that the manufacturers needed to be relieved of liability for their products. The nation's public debate about medical care seldom focuses on the dark side of all such interventions: that some are inevitably harmed, even die. Thanks to the vaccine manufacturers, the public got an unfocused crash course in the hazards of what was previously regarded as the most benign of all medical procedures, a vaccination.

More and more influential voices of dissent were heard in the scientific and medical community. Some of these experts weren't consulted in the rapid decision to get vaccine production into full gear. Others were consulted, at least informally, and had not spoken out when it mattered, or had spoken so tentatively that their voices were not heard.

When the immunizations actually began, the whole enterprise had become so controversial that events that otherwise might have passed unnoticed became instant national news. In Pennsylvania, three elderly individuals with existing heart problems died soon after getting their flu shots. Was the vaccine contaminated? This did not prove to be the case. Finally the program ground entirely to a halt by the possibility, later established in fact, that flu immunization increased by a factor of eight the risk of paralysis through the rare Guillian-Barré syndrome.

Because no swine flu epidemic occurred, the final and perhaps most important failure of the program almost entirely escaped public notice. The manufacturers had not even come close to producing enough vaccine in time. The 1957 pandemic struck right at the beginning of the flu season—in October—and swept across the country in three weeks. By that time in 1976, less than 1 percent of the population had been immunized, a worse performance than in a normal flu year. The final "deadline" for producing the necessary 200 million doses was finally set for February 15, 1977. With two additional weeks required to achieve immunity, vaccination would have amounted to little more than closing the barn door after the horse got out—or never arrived.

Lessons were learned, although it was by no means clear whether most of the precedents set were good ones. Gerald Ford lost the presidency, and the swine flu episode undoubtedly contributed. After President Carter took office, his secretary of Health, Education and Welfare, Joseph Califano, sent the health community an unmistakable message. Califano removed Sencer, the director who came up through the ranks, and replaced him with a political appointee whose first loyalty would be to the president. To those who follow such nuances, it was a clear message that nobody at CDC was ever again going to point a gun, political or otherwise, at the president of the United States.

At CDC an era of greater caution prevails. The CDC has taken a back seat to the National Institutes of Health in the struggle to combat AIDS, the most dangerous infectious disease threat of the postwar period. Alan Kendal, who now heads the influenza branch of CDC, was asked what lessons for future flu crises had been learned from the swine flu episode. He responded that he would be very careful to seek the broadest possible consensus before taking action. That, perhaps, is the correct political lesson of the swine flu episode, but it seems clear that no one has yet taught that kind of patience to the influenza virus.

The real lesson of the swine flu episode has largely escaped the notice of both the professionals and the public. The message, loud and clear, is that three times since World War II the United States has tried to confront the threat of influenza. All three times the flu won. The next big threat from influenza could come at any time: in the next week, next month or next decade. Unless there is a serious reassessment and a major standby plan already in place, it appears nearly certain that the flu will emerge victorious once again. And next time the cost may not be measured in scientific embarrassment, injured reputations and high-level jobs lost. The costs of still another failure will be measured in thousands of lives unnecessarily lost, life expectancy needlessly reduced. A little-noticed episode in 1983, when the swine flu episode was mostly forgotten, provides a dramatic illustration of that point.

Doctor Robert J. Eckroad had already been tracking the mildest of influenza A epidemics as it swept through the farming country of Lancaster County, Pennsylvania, beginning in April. Eckroad hadn't seen much flu in his area for some time, so he watched the progress with interest. The viruses were isolated and typed in his laboratory at the University of Pennsylvania in Kennett Square.

Then, in October of 1983, a mild strain of influenza A, without warning, mutated into a lethal killer with a mortality rate of 50 to 90 percent. It made the 1918 influenza look like a mild disease. One factor made this a particular shock: this was not a case of genetic shift that suddenly enabled the virus to overcome immune defenses. This strain was identical with the benign strain that had been circulating through the area for the past few months. Except now, because of a single point mutation in the HA protein spike, it was now a killer virus.

Fortunately for the human race, this influenza A virus strain infected only the poultry flocks of Pennsylvania and Virginia. Even among birds the costs were extremely high: 17 million birds quickly slaughtered to contain the lethal strain of avian influenza, a strain fortunately never seen in humans.

Edwin Kilbourne, perhaps the nation's leading authority on the genetic structure of the influenza virus, was asked if a similar point mutation could occur in human strains:

"It could," he said.

So the dice game continues. Like it or not, mankind steps up to the table to wager lives in a game in which someone else made the rules, and previous performance hardly inspires confidence.

It is foolish to ignore the possibility that the world of microscopic life-forms may one day reclaim the gains in life expectancy that were wrested from its grasp over the past century and a half. Should such a disaster occur, influenza remains not only the best-documented case study, but also an important direct threat. Further cautionary lessons can be learned, however, from examining what happened when a different and unknown viral invader of great potential menace suddenly appeared.

CHAPTER SIX

A VIRUS EMERGES

An onlooker might have thought that a science fiction movie was being filmed. In the Washington, D.C., suburb of Reston, Virginia, eight men and women had gathered outside a nondescript one-story brick building near a shopping center. They put on bright orange plastic jump suits with a broad vertical black stripe down the middle, and clear plastic helmets. Thus equipped, each turned a switch on a boxlike unit on the belt, and a fan began to whir quietly and the suit inflated, making them look like an army of identical, clumsy orange snowmen. They were wearing positive-pressure suits, designed so that no moisture droplet, dust speck or viral particle could be admitted without being captured as it passed through a high-efficiency particulate aerosol filter. Even if someone accidentally snagged the suit while working inside the brick building, the positive pressure in the suit would protect them because the air would leak out, not seep in.

They had assembled an impressive array of equipment. There were hypodermic syringes and bottles filled with a rapidly lethal poison mixed with barbiturates. They had enormous quantities of plastic bags and boxes. Many carried cylindrical containers with hand pumps and a hose that looked something like an overgrown version of a garden sprayer for insecticides. The orange snowmen worked for the United States Army Medical Research Institute of Infectious Disease. They were based at the former military center for biological warfare at Fort Detrick, Maryland, located 27 miles north of Washington. It was late December 1989, and this was no drill.

The building housed a biomedical research firm called Hazelton Research Products. Confined in special isolation cages inside were more than 400 macaque monkeys that had been imported from the Philippines over the past three months and then quarantined for observation. They were the first target for the invading biomedical SWAT team. All the monkeys were killed with an injection. The bodies were placed in double-sealed pouches and taken to Fort Detrick. There, in a special containment facility, tissue samples were taken from each. The bodies were sterilized in a high-pressure steam autoclave. To be absolutely certain, this procedure was repeated again. Only then would the remains be removed from the containment building and incinerated.

Back in Reston, the team spent days on decontamination. Practically every portable object was removed and placed in a plastic bag. The bag was sprayed with chlorine bleach, and then placed in still another bag. This too was sprayed. The bags were deposited in special contaminated-material carriers dubbed "hatboxes" because of their similarity to the containers for ladies' fancy headgear. The hatboxes were also sealed and sprayed. Then the material was removed to Fort Detrick and incinerated. Every floor, wall, ceiling, shelf, window and door was scrubbed with bleach. The whole building was fumigated with an aerosol variant of formaldehyde. Insofar as possible, all living matter was eradicated, everything from the size of a medium-sized monkey right down to stringy-looking viral particles visible only when magnified ten thousand times in an electron microscope.

It would be an understatement to say that both civilian and military medical authorities were concerned about what had unexpectedly gotten loose inside the building in Reston, Virginia. A few days earlier they had identified a virus so rare that only three previous outbreaks had ever been reported. Remarkably little was known about it, except for one striking characteristic. In the first recorded incident, 88 percent of those infected soon died of massive internal hemorrhaging, making it one of the most lethal viruses known to man. It was named Ebola, after the picturesque river in central Africa where the first terrifying outbreak occurred in 1976.

A rare African virus relates more directly to human life expectancy than might be immediately apparent. The preceding chapters have outlined the major dimensions of a changing relationship with microscopic life-forms that constitutes the most important factor regulating the human lifespan. A journey that began by peering into the mists of earliest human history will now conclude at the opposite boundary, by considering the future possibilities of that relationship. This chapter will seek to explore the future as it is reflected in a detailed account of a modern-day confrontation with a dangerous virus. It is certain that the next major encounter with an unknown disease will differ from the episode reported here. But it should illuminate many key features of what may lie ahead.

The extreme nature of the response in Reston, Virginia, was based primarily on what had occurred in the first known outbreak of Ebola. Those events were etched into the collective memory of those responsible for managing the biological crisis in Reston.

In the deepest and most remote heart of equatorial Africa lies the Bumba Zone of Zaire. It is a land of dense, primeval jungle dotted with tiny villages of mud and wattle huts. On August 26, 1976, a 44-year-old teacher in the Yambuku mission school checked into the mission hospital with a fever following a tour through the neighboring areas. He was diagnosed with malaria, given an injection of chloroquine, and sent home.

The 120-bed Yambuku Hospital had been operated by Catholic missionaries from Belgium since 1935, a last vestige of the colonial days when Zaire was called the Belgian Congo. It provided medical care for 60,000 inhabitants of the surrounding area, and was so well known and widely patronized that the outpatient clinic might see 6,000 patients from hundreds of tiny villages in a single month. It had a staff of 17.

Just a few days later, on September 1, the teacher was back in the hospital with a raging fever. A week later he died of massive gastrointestinal bleeding. By that time there were nine more cases of fever, headache, and finally severe bleeding and death. By the end of the month, the Yambuku Mission Hospital was closed entirely after 11 of the 17 health-care workers had died.

One of the surviving nurses, a Catholic nun from Belgium, was admitted to Ngaliema Hospital in Kinshasa, the capital of Zaire. Soon she also died. Next the two Kinshasa nurses who had cared for her during her nine-day illness also died. None of the physicians who attended these cases had ever seen a disease like this before. Panic ensued. The whole staff of the hospital ward where the three nurses had died was quarantined, along with others who had close contact with the nurses. The whole Bumba region was isolated, with transportation and services abruptly severed. Since the mysterious disease had already reached Kinshasa, European air lines were considering terminating their service. Out went an international call for medical help.

In medical circles there had been quiet discussion of the mainly theoretical problem of "emerging viruses." Some thoughtful researchers were concerned that humanity might suddenly be assaulted either by a benign virus that suddenly mutated into more virulent form, or by an already-lethal invader that was lurking undetected in some remote corner of the world, waiting for a golden opportunity. Here, in Zaire, was apparently the real thing, a lethal, previously unknown disease. From around the world literally hundreds of physicians, virologists and other researchers swiftly gathered in Kinshasa to do battle with this unknown peril.

One of the first to arrive was a world authority on rare tropical viruses named Karl M. Johnson. He headed the federal Centers for Disease Control's unit that studied exotic and little-known viruses, called the special pathogens branch. By the time Johnson got to Kinshasa, the virus had already been identified in his own laboratory back at CDC headquarters in Atlanta and in two laboratories in Europe. It was brand new, but a fairly close relative of the virus called Marburg, which was named after the German city where seven laboratory workers had died after working with the virus-infected tissues of African green monkeys. With the electron microscope, the Ebola virus particles looked something like pretzels of varying length.

When Johnson reached Kinshasa no one had yet answered the question upon which literally millions of lives might depend. "What we didn't know was how this one was being transmitted. If you had an agent that might be spread by the respiratory route then we might be facing the Andromeda strain. For a period of about two or three weeks, everyone held their breath."

The fictional brush with doomsday portrayed in *The Andromeda*

Strain did not occur in modern-day Zaire. Evidence accumulated that the virus could not be transmitted except through close personal contact or blood.

But initially, this reassuring fact was not known to Johnson or his medical colleagues, who were fanning out through the African jungle in pursuit of this new predator of man. One physician in the field, working for Johnson in the special pathogens branch of CDC, was a round-faced, youthful specialist in rare viruses named Joseph McCormick. For him, being buried in the jungle of Zaire was like coming home.

To McCormick fell the job of traversing seven hundred miles of untamed jungle—traveling from the Bumba Zone across the border into a remote corner of the Sudan where another Ebola outbreak had been reported at about the same time. In McCormick's life, it was almost a full circle, because this was the very place where his interest in medicine had been first inspired. After college, McCormick had joined the Peace Corps and had been posted to Zaire as a schoolteacher in another Belgian mission. He had been there when Patrice Lumumba had driven the country into revolutionary chaos, so he did little teaching. But he was also handy, and devoted much of his spare time to rebuilding the mission hospital, which had been wrecked in the conflict. Appreciative hospital doctors started taking him on rounds, and when he finally left Africa, he knew medicine was his calling.

Now he was back, driving a Land Rover, and heading toward the Sudan. He spoke French, the predominant European language, and even some Lingala and Krio, two local languages. Armed with an old Michelin map he drove down jungle paths, fording rivers with the Land Rover tied to planks lashed across two dugouts. He was the first Westerner to reach Nzara, the remote epidemic site in the Sudan. Unfortunately there was not much to see. The epidemic had struck more than two months earlier, and practically all the victims were dead. But he took samples, interviewed methodically, and then headed back to Zaire.

The international team, meanwhile, had learned everything it could about this strange new Ebola virus. They had interviewed 34,000 families with 280,000 members in 550 villages. They confirmed 318 cases of Ebola of whom only 38 survived. The breakthrough was tracking down the primary means by which the disease had initially spread. It was a vivid demonstration that the blessings of modern medicine can, under some conditions, become a deadly curse.

It was the practice of the hospital staff in Yambuku to provide only five syringes and needles for each day's outpatient population, which could number hundreds of individuals. The needles were not cleaned between uses. A majority of the Ebola cases had been outpatients at the hospital; the remainder had had extremely close personal contact with the ailing victim, mostly spouses and children. No one who got Ebola through contaminated needles survived. So while this was a very nasty bug, it was reassuring to learn that it was relatively hard to transmit. It moved from person to person more readily than AIDS, but nothing like the lightning speed of transmission seen in respiratory viruses like those that cause measles and flu.

On the other hand, once inside the body Ebola had the capacity to multiply with astonishing rapidity. Karl Johnson remembered seeing samples in which 10 million viral particles could be found in a single milliliter, or about a third of an ounce of blood.

One extremely important mystery remains unsolved. Where, in nature, does Ebola hide? What animals are its natural hosts? Without a regular succession of hosts in which to replicate, the virus would quickly face extinction. How did the first humans become infected? The researchers studied the ground-up remains of 818 bedbugs without finding a trace of the virus. Nor was any evidence of Ebola found in 3 species of mosquitoes, 10 pigs, 7 bats, 30 squirrels, 30 rats and 6 monkeys. They simply could not find the natural lair of the deadly Ebola.

The Zairean outbreak ultimately became a moderately famous episode in the annals of medicine, and in some retellings, the story ends on a note of technological triumph, as the band of experts assembled from around the world bottled up and controlled this new menace.

But as Karl Johnson, who headed the World Health Organization team, remembers it, nothing of the kind ever happened.

"It fundamentally died a natural death," he said. "When the hospital didn't work anymore, and there were no more needles and syringes transmitting the disease directly, the epidemic began to wane on its own account.

"They also began to figure out in the villages that if somebody died, the ones who were getting the disease were among those completely responsible for the feeding and care of the person while alive.

"They went back to their ancient way of dealing with outbreaks of lethal disease, which was that you suspend the cultural rules about caring for people and about funerals. You put the sick person in a hut. You put food and water in the door. If the person walks out someday, or crawls out, that's fine. If not, you burn the hut."

Over the intervening years little more was learned about the Ebola virus. McCormick returned to monitor another small outbreak in the Sudan in 1979, but again the spread of the disease halted without intervention. To those who study the relationship between humans and disease, Ebola became a dramatic example of the larger problem of emerging viruses. They are described as *emerging* rather than *new* viruses because they are just as much a product of gradual evolution as are other living things. Nothing springs to life spontaneously. Viruses may suddenly find new hosts, invade new kinds of specialized cells, or acquire or lose virulence. But they had to have descended from some predecessor or conceivably combined the genetic material from two. But, always, hiding in some biological niche somewhere are the precursors of what might tomorrow become new and lethal diseases.

Improving our understanding of how viruses emerge has become more urgent since a virus infecting African monkeys leaped to humans 20 to 40 years ago. It had already affected millions of humans before it was identified as the virus that causes AIDS. Meanwhile, an important question about Ebola remains unanswered.

Except in the contaminated needle cases, no one could identify specifically how the virus entered the body. The official description— through close personal contact—covered a multitude of possible routes of transmission. Nor was serious progress made in identifying the natural host for this disease. Monkeys were the key suspect, since they carried the related Marburg virus. But despite searching the jungles, no trace of Ebola antibodies could be found in African monkeys. And when introduced into laboratory monkeys, it invariably killed them, making it unlikely that this was the natural host. A virus that kills its host so quickly soon runs out of hosts, and extinguishes itself.

Other more pressing health concerns would command the medical research dollars. Also, Ebola was so dangerous that there were only two places in the entire medical research establishment of the United States with adequate safety precautions. One was the CDC's own P-4 containment facility in Atlanta. The other was the Army's similar facility sited at the former biological warfare lab at Fort Detrick, Maryland. At the Army medical research facility at Fort Detrick, rare tropical viruses were studied by a Cornell University-trained physician and microbiologist named Peter B. Jahrling.

It was only for the most obscure of reasons that in late 1989 Peter Jahrling happened to be examining tissue samples from Asian monkeys. They had been sent from the Hazelton Research Products facility in Reston, Virginia, which housed up to 500 recently imported primates destined for use in medical and other research. To protect against disease that might spread to humans, the monkeys were quarantined for 45 days after entering the United States. Near the end of the quarantine period for a group of 100 macaque monkeys from the Philippines, the animals began to die in unusual numbers. Jahrling had become known in the tight-knit community that worked with primates as an expert in a rare virus called simian hemorrhagic fever. While capable of devastating a primate community, especially in captivity, it was harmless to humans. The veterinarian at Hazelton, Dan Dalgard, suspected that was what was killing his macaques, and asked Jahrling to help.

The initial challenge in identifying any virus is to find a laboratory culture of living cells in which it will grow. Simian hemorrhagic fever virus had proved particularly difficult, but could be coaxed to multiply slowly in a culture of kidney cells from rhesus monkeys.

One day in November 1989, Jahrling's technician, Joan Rhoderick, noticed something quite unusual. They had finished three of the four samples, and had in each case found the characteristic spherical particles of simian hemorrhagic fever. But in the last of the flasks, something was rapidly destroying the kidney cells, hardly the performance expected from the hard-to-grow simian hemorrhagic fever virus. Virologists call this cytopathic effect or CPE. But rampaging viruses are not invariably the culprit. Often bacterial or fungal contamination from the air can also kill off the cell cultures.

Rhoderick showed the flask to Jahrling. He sniffed it for evidence of contamination. Nothing seemed amiss. Rhoderick sniffed it, too, and noticed no telltale odors. That would have been the end of it had not Tom Geisberg, a young technician, volunteered to exercise his newly learned skills with the electron microscope to find out why this strain of simian hemorrhagic fever was so destructive. Later that day, Geisberg put the 10,000-magnification photograph in front of Jahrling, without comment.

"This is *not* funny," said Jahrling. It showed dozens of slender, filamentous viral particles. An additional test confirmed his worst fears. They had been sniffing a flask in an open laboratory that contained one of the deadliest viruses known to man. It was unlikely the virus could escape from the P-3 laboratory in which they were working, but they had been personally exposed. It seemed utterly impossible, but it was the Ebola virus.

Jahrling will never forget the moment: "I should know better. I do know better. When you get an unknown sample you treat it like an unknown sample."

Fort Detrick has a special hospital suite that includes the most elaborate protection against the transmission of deadly disease of any facility in the world. And as Jahrling looked at the electron micrograph of the Ebola particles, he considered immediately confining himself and the technician to the facility. Then, faced with an extraordinary and unexpected experimental result, he did what microbiologists the world over do almost without exception: repeat the experiment on the assumption that some kind of weird mistake has been made. This required four more nervous days of painstaking laboratory work. The initial results were no fluke.

"This is *not* funny."

This time, the speaker of these now familiar words was General Philip Russell, commander of the Army Research Institute at Fort Detrick. Jahrling had just told him that they had identified the Ebola virus at an animal facility in Reston, Virginia. Russell picked up the telephone and called CDC in Atlanta, where he reached Frederick A. Murphy, director of the Center for Infectious Diseases. The next flight leaving Atlanta for

Washington, D.C., carried Fred Murphy and the CDC's Ebola expert, Joseph McCormick, who had succeeded Karl Johnson as branch chief.

Whatever happened next was not going to be quietly managed by disease professionals. A disease as lethal and exotic as the Ebola virus found in the United States offered all the necessary ingredients for a genuine, full-scale, three-ring media circus. A suburban newspaper had already begun asking questions. The CDC in particular would be required to play the role of the confident professionals in the full glare of media scrutiny while handling the outbreak of a lethal disease about which, in fact, they knew little. And to start, all they had was the tissue sample of one deceased macaque monkey in Hazelton's room F. Conceivably there was no hazard here at all.

On the evening of November 29, 1989, members of the Virginia health department, the CDC and the Army huddled at Fort Detrick to make a plan of action. Given the many players, large number of unknowns, and the potential for overkill, underkill and overlooking some minor factor that would later prove to be of paramount importance, their plan was a model of cool, rational response.

A low-key statement was issued to the news media. It revealed that the Ebola virus had been tentatively identified in the primate population at Hazelton, and little else. The next problem was to identify who might be already infected with the Ebola virus. The most obvious candidates were those with direct or indirect contact with the infected monkeys. That put the animal handlers and the vets at Hazelton in the highest risk category. Those with other jobs at the facility were at medium risk. And finally there were the spouses, families and others in close contact with those who worked with the monkeys. Approximately 40 to 50 persons in all composed the group most likely to get the disease. All were put under daily medical surveillance—a procedure that primarily involved taking their temperature daily, and reporting it to an Epidemiological Intelligence Service officer assigned to keep score. Periodic blood samples would be scrutinized for telltale evidence of antibodies to Ebola.

If someone did get sick, the team was soon prepared: from Atlanta the CDC airlifted a mobile virus laboratory. At nearby Fairfax Hospital, they identified a special suite where patients could be isolated. And the CDC had already developed hospital guidelines to prevent nursing and medical personnel from getting the disease. During the outbreaks in Zaire, the Sudan, and Marburg, Germany, nurses or other attending personnel had been infected.

The next priority was to prevent further spread of the disease. Part of the problem was automatically solved because the macaque monkeys were already in quarantine—the payoff for a required precaution. All that was required was to tighten the isolation. Animal handlers would wear respirators and protective suits while in contact with the monkeys. Tighter procedures would be instituted to prevent spread between animals. That meant that if Ebola was going to escape into the United States population, it would likely do so through the approximately 40 people who might be already infected but had no symptoms yet. In the Zaire outbreak, the incubation period ranged from 3 to 21 days. This raised the first serious issue on which opinion was initially divided. To guarantee no further spread of Ebola into the human population, should the people at risk be quarantined? Right there at Fort Detrick was the functional equivalent of a minimum security prison which could accommodate them. Should they use it?

This policy of seemingly greatest caution was not without its own risks. Literally locking up 40 to 50 people for three weeks would make the episode a national sensation, and could, argued some CDC officials, create a public panic. And if nobody got sick they might look foolish.

One of the loudest voices for a policy of minimum action was Ebola veteran McCormick, who was not fully convinced there was a real crisis at all. If the virus were so lethal, he reasoned, humans would already be ill.

The Army's Jahrling, however, was not so sure. "All known Ebola isolated had been virulent to humans and we had no reason to suppose this might be different," he said.

One critical question could not be immediately answered. How did the Reston monkeys become infected in the first place? It was not hard to imagine that Ebola might be harbored by some species of African monkey that had never been tested. But this disease was coming from Asia. The working hypothesis, therefore, was that these Philippine monkeys had somehow become infected by African animals while being transported to Reston, Virginia. Finding the original source of infection was exactly the kind of medical detective work for which the Epidemiological Intelligence Service was justly famous, and within hours, the EIS was tracing the route of the shipment.

The monkeys had been trucked to Reston from Kennedy Airport on Long Island, the port of entry for a majority of the 20,000 monkeys imported into the United States each year. Steve Ostrow, the director of the EIS, headed for New York. There Ostrow discovered the flood of incoming animals was not tightly quarantined, creating a multitude of possible sources of cross-infection. But this shipment of 100 monkeys had been quickly unloaded from the aircraft and immediately put on trucks. They didn't become infected at JFK.

The flight had arrived from the busiest and most important animal transshipment point in the world: Amsterdam. The World Health Organization would cooperate. From its Geneva headquarters, two investigators were dispatched to Amsterdam to inquire. They were joined by a CDC expert, who flew in from Atlanta.

In Amsterdam, it was learned that the animal port was tightly organized, and excellent records were kept. While in Amsterdam, the Reston monkeys had indeed been in contact with African primates. Specifically, they might have been infected by one gibbon or one red-tailed monkey, both of which had been recently captured in Ghana. Now the CDC had to find these two monkeys.

Within a few days' time, the CDC had traced them to a private zoo in Mexico City. A cooperating veterinarian was recruited to visit the zoo. He found the monkeys were alive and well, and shipped blood samples to Atlanta. There was no trace of Ebola virus antibodies.

Meanwhile, back in Reston, Virginia, the Ebola virus continued to spread. Although a single tissue sample had triggered the entire crisis, Jahrling's laboratory soon had identified five more cases. More disturbing still, despite strict isolation procedures, the Ebola had escaped from room F, and now was sweeping through an entirely different shipment of monkeys.

Then one morning a 50-year-old animal handler vomited and fell ill. He had earlier been bitten by one of the monkeys in room F. Veterinarian Dan Dalgard took his temperature: 101.5 degrees Fahrenheit. It was possible that the Ebola had now moved to humans. This was not exactly a private medical crisis. The press corps was camped out at Hazelton and saw the handler, dressed in a protective suit, get sick, and then be carried away in an ambulance, siren screaming. He was placed in the previously prepared room at Fairfax Hospital for observation. And on that day, December 4, 1989, it was decided that all the monkeys should be killed and the entire Reston facility decontaminated. The orange-suited Army went to work.

As the year drew to a close it looked like the Ebola crisis might be over. The monkeys were dead. The animal handler did not develop Ebola, nor did anyone else at Hazelton Research Products. By the end of December blood tests of the population at risk showed no trace of Ebola antibodies. So no one died, no one got sick, no one even had a serious enough exposure to trigger a response from the body's immune defenses. At CDC headquarters, consideration was given to stricter controls over primate imports—even a temporary embargo, but no action was taken.

It looked like the Ebola crisis was over, a textbook exercise in disease control. Inevitably, there were unanswered questions. Where did the disease come from? Was this strain less virulent to humans, or was no one sufficiently exposed for infection to occur? The most critical observer might have concluded that a good system performed well. The CDC-required quarantine for primate imports had worked as expected. Clear and decisive action had contained the outbreak. A varied cast had worked smoothly together. It looked like here was a system that could protect the country from such emerging viruses. It would take only a few more weeks to demonstrate that was hardly the case.

Just six weeks later, it appeared that a major biological disaster might be about to occur. Once again, numerous cases of Ebola were being detected, except this time the outbreak was not limited to a single quarantine facility: the disease was being found among primates shipped to at least three states: Texas, Pennsylvania and Virginia. Since the first outbreak in Zaire, virologists had breathed a sigh of relief because there seemed to be no evidence that Ebola could be transmitted by the respiratory route. As the disease spread rapidly among primates, the evidence mounted that this variety of Ebola was almost surely transmitted through the air and entered the respiratory system. Finally, the new, wider outbreak was going to settle a vital question left unanswered in the preceding episode. No cases in humans had been observed, not even the telltale evidence of elevated antibodies, which would signal that infection had occurred but that the body's immune defenses had triumphed. Was this new strain unlike all other known strains of Ebola, and simply not a serious threat to humans? Or had no one been exposed? This time there was no doubt that several humans had been directly exposed.

How, in just a few weeks' time, was apparent success transformed into a possible disaster? Every disease episode leaves behind many unanswered questions, some of which prove more important than others. In this case, a global investigation had failed to identify the source of the disease. No one knew for sure how the virus had initially entered the United States, except that it involved imported macaque monkeys. Therefore, no action was taken, although a temporary import ban was considered. With the door left open and unattended, diseased animals now entered the country in greater numbers. And as the realization dawned, the most agonizing question was whether someone was going to die as a result of this oversight. And if someone did, there was little doubt about the leading candidate: his name was Tiny Meriman, and he worked as an animal handler at the same Reston, Virginia, facility where the first outbreak had occurred.

Following the massive decontamination effort, Hazelton Research Products had resumed macaque imports in January, and two shipments of monkeys arrived without incident. In the early weeks of the quarantine period the animals were well. At the end of the month a third shipment arrived, 200 animals from the same exporter in the Philippines that had long been Hazelton's prime supplier. Half the animals went to Texas, the other half to Reston. It was soon clear to Dan Dalgard, the Hazelton veterinarian, that the animals were getting sick and dying even more rapidly than in the December outbreak.

At Hazelton, the handlers performed the animal version of an autopsy on the dead monkeys to obtain tissue samples for further testing. In the first week of February there were a large number of dead animals requiring this procedure. During one of these autopsies, Tiny Meriman had both hands in the abdominal cavity attempting to obtain a sample of the liver. One hand slipped and he cut it, puncturing the latex gloves he was wearing.

Fort Detrick quickly confirmed two facts: the monkeys were indeed

dying of Ebola. And the liver that Meriman was removing was loaded
with the virus. In 3 to 21 days' time, the incubation period of Ebola,
everyone would know whether or not this strain of Ebola was dangerous
to humans. So concerned was the CDC that a young physician and
Epidemiological Intelligence Service officer was dispatched to monitor
Tiny Meriman's health.

The incubation period passed, and Meriman did not get even mildly
ill. He had, however, been infected. A blood sample showed that millions upon millions of antibodies specific to Ebola were circulating.
They could only have been produced in this quantity if the immune
system had specifically identified this invader, triggering the rapid multiplication of the white blood cells capable of manufacturing this particular, unique antibody.

Meriman was not the only case. Four more workers at the Reston
facility showed a major antibody response—none had cut themselves or
otherwise been so closely exposed. CDC expanded the search for Ebola
cases and found 42 persons with similarly elevated antibodies among
those who had worked with primates. The CDC even found a case right
at its own headquarters, an animal handler who had had no contact with
primates for almost two years.

This was the picture as the facts finally came into focus: this virus had
entered the United States through more routes and infected more people than anyone had suspected. Unlike the African strains, it was much
more contagious, capable of transmission by the respiratory route. Unlike the African strains, which killed up to 88 percent of those infected,
this strain didn't even make a single person mildly ill. The United States
had been incredibly lucky.

The disease profile of what came to be called the Reston strain proved
so unlike the African variants that a new family of viruses was created:
filoviruses. It included the African Ebola, the deadly Marburg, and the
apparently harmless Reston strain. No one had any idea why the Reston
strain did not cause disease in humans. Under the electron microscope
the particles of all three viruses appeared similar. All the strains reacted
to some of the same antibodies, but not perfectly, indicating that some
features of the viruses were different.

The CDC suspended the importation of all primates for 16 months,
during which it developed new procedures for testing and handling the

animals. The source of the Reston, Texas and Pennsylvania outbreaks was ultimately traced to a single facility of a single shipper in the Philippines.

Nature had rolled the dice. And this time it was an emerging virus that proved to be much more infectious than related strains, but much less lethal. Nobody could possibly know what the next roll of the dice might bring.

Ten years after the first Ebola outbreak in Zaire, Joe McCormick and an international group of colleagues decided to reexamine the hundreds of samples of blood serum collected in the field and stored since then in a freezer at CDC. This time they searched for early evidence of a different emerging virus. To their surprise they found that 0.8 percent of the samples tested positive for the AIDS virus. It had been prevalent in Africa at least seven years before the virus was first isolated by French researcher Luc Montagnier in 1983. The researchers also returned to the Bumba Zone to collect 388 new samples. The AIDS infection rate was still 0.8 percent. Finally, they tested the blood of 283 female prostitutes in larger towns. This time 11 percent were already infected with AIDS. It was an arresting example of how a virus emerges.

The AIDS virus, it is now clear, was present in the isolated villages of central Africa, although, if this sample is an indication, at a very low rate of infection. An occasional premature death would not have attracted undue attention in a region where life expectancy was short, premature death commonplace and medical attention rudimentary. (In fact, three of the five subjects found infected in 1976 blood samples were dead 10 years later.) One of the leading students of the origin of AIDS, Gerald Meyers of Brookhaven National Laboratory, believes that AIDS began in Africa 20 to 40 years ago. A related disease of primates—simian immunodeficiency virus—changed just enough to survive in humans.

In any event, the mutation in the AIDS virus probably was not sufficient itself to trigger a global epidemic. It is extremely difficult to transmit, and its latency period of many years was likely an evolutionary response of the virus that enabled it to survive. If it killed quickly, like Ebola, it would have died out before it could spread to others. AIDS spread around the globe because changes in human behavior suddenly opened new avenues for transmission. The breakdown of traditional customs in Africa promoted the spread; a global transportation system created the opportunity for a small foothold in Europe. Then the promiscuous sexual practices of the American gay community created the perfect conditions for an enormous outbreak.

AIDS remains a major, untamed peril to human life. Like many viruses, the AIDS virus is a single strand of RNA, and therefore capable of rapid mutation. A second characteristic multiplies its menace by many times. It includes the instructions for an enzyme called reverse transcriptase. This allows the single strand of RNA to be translated into double-stranded DNA, which integrates itself into the genetic code of human white blood cells, concealed out of sight, multiplying when the white blood cells multiply. Finally it destroys one class of white blood cells, called CD4 cells, through an unknown mechanism. This leaves the door open to the entire constellation of bacterial and viral invaders.

Vaccine development is severely handicapped by two features of the AIDS virus. Like herpes and CMV it can lurk, latent and concealed from antibodies, inside living cells, multiplying as they multiply. Second, since there are no long-term AIDS survivors, there is no known successful immune response. How can attenuated or inactivated virus be used to provoke a successful immune response when there is no evidence that such an immune response has ever occurred? A successful vaccine will depend on advances in scientific knowledge that will enable development of a vaccine that creates immune response in humans that has never occurred naturally.★

AIDS and Ebola are the most spectacular examples, but they are by no means the only examples of emerging viruses and other diseases of which we have become newly aware.

Most "new" diseases prove to have existed for decades, if not centuries. The outbreak of Legionnaires' disease in a Philadelphia hotel proved to be caused by a common bacterium that grew in practically any body of water—but not in laboratory cultures traditionally used to study them. Sometimes the infectious agent has been identified, but its disease-causing capacity not fully understood. For example, ulcers, once thought

---

★This brief examination of AIDS is not a reflection of its importance, which cannot be overstated, but because so much information is readily available from other sources.

to be caused by stress and other behavioral factors, may be a result of bacterial infection by *Campylobacter priori,* a well-known intestinal microbe.

Sometimes there are new "diseases" without any known causal agent. The most publicized is chronic fatigue syndrome, or the so-called yuppie flu. Victims are so debilitated they are unable to work for months, and sometimes years. But no disease-causing agent has ever been identified. One possibility is an elusive and rare combination of circumstances. An example is Reye's Syndrome which once caused several hundred cases of severe kidney disease in children each year, and was frequently fatal. The syndrome was convincingly established as a rare complication of taking aspirin in the presence of chickenpox or influenza. In another example, for many decades thousands suffered from the unexplained symptoms of fatigue, loss of appetite and malaise. It was later identified as chronic infection by the hepatitis B virus.

Viruses have also emerged from a phenomenon that might be described as naturally occurring genetic engineering. In one documented case a new virus causing inflammation of the brain tissue of horses contained features from two separate and distinct equine viruses.

A growing but difficult-to-assess threat is the possibility of diseases created by accidental or deliberate genetic engineering. The debate about the safety and regulation of genetic engineering is following a cycle similar to that involving nuclear safety regulation. The industry, fearful of being hamstrung by outside regulation, has assured the public that what they're doing is perfectly safe. Critics have mixed genuine concerns with blind fear of the unknown. Evidence is already emerging that genetic engineering is not as safe as the industry maintains. There are already at least two genetic engineering accidents on the public record.

In 1988 the CDC began investigating a strange series of cases of a rare and painful blood disorder called eosinophilia-myalgia syndrome. Ultimately the problem was traced to contaminated supplies of an amino acid called L-tryptophan manufactured by a Japanese company and sold as an over-the-counter sedative. In the process of inserting the gene to manufacture the amino acid into *E. coli* bacteria something went wrong and the resulting product caused disease.

In 1991 a trial of a possible AIDS vaccine in Zaire was abruptly halted because of a whole series of irregularities. The concept of the vaccine was ingenious. A gene resembling a key surface protein of the AIDS virus was grafted onto the DNA of the cowpox virus. The idea was that in developing immunity to the cowpox virus, the body would also produce antibodies to a key component of the AIDS virus at the same time. Unfortunately not all the genetically engineered cowpox virus was inactivated. It might have been harmless to a normal healthy volunteer, but it proved fatal to immunocompromised AIDS patients. The approach did not work, and the National Institutes of Health Office of Scientific Integrity concluded that the whole experiment was unethical research on subjects whose prior consent had not been obtained. Although this is the only publicly known accident with genetically engineered viruses, they are routinely altered and used as carriers to insert genetic material into cells.

In addition to genetic engineering accidents, there is the possibility of deliberate introduction of newly created diseases through biological warfare. As a military weapon it has many drawbacks. The most important are that the effects are unpredictable and the victims might be one's own population rather than an adversary. For this and ethical reasons, the major world powers have disavowed biological warfare and opened their remaining research facilities to international inspection.

While uncontrolled and unpredictable in its effects, biological warfare is nevertheless the cheapest and most readily obtained method of mass destruction. Biological weapons could be created, from the open scientific literature, by a bright postdoctoral fellow in microbiology using materials readily available by mail order from a biological supply house.

A virus may emerge because it acquires a new host animal or because a vector through which it travels acquires new opportunities to expand its territory. A virus carried by the Asian striped field mouse causes 100,000 cases of hemorrhagic fever a year in China. A close relative of the virus is able to survive in the principal urban rat species, *Rattus rattus*. As a result, this virus, which causes Seoul hemorrhagic fever, has spread rapidly around the world. A recent study of inner city rats in Baltimore found 64 percent had antibodies to Seoul hemorrhagic fever.

. . .

From Samuel Preston's analysis of factors that might increase life expectancy, we saw earlier that future gains from the elimination of infectious disease as a cause of death will be relatively small—on the order of two years. The more serious possibility remains that the gains of the past 20 to 40 years might be reversed by an emerging virus or other disease. The preceding chapters have sought to make clear that the relationship has been transformed by the ascendancy of modern science, but it has hardly been abolished. What, then, are the current strengths and weaknesses of human defenses?

Medical and biological technology have brought the obvious towering strengths. Most bacterial disease can be readily defeated today, and more is being learned about the much more difficult problem of viruses. A peaceful, prosperous society has brought the healthiest, most robust populations the world has ever known. Sanitation, protected water supplies, and high standards of personal hygiene have closed off—or at least narrowed—many of the avenues of attack. A worldwide epidemiological network exists to identify and neutralize disease threats.

But modern industrialized society also brings important new vulnerabilities. The increasingly dense mass of humanity makes a rich target for disease. As the historian William McNeill puts it, "There is a magnificent feeding ground out there with millions and millions of bodies." An efficient network of air and sea transportation cements the world into one interrelated system. It also provides ideal vehicles for the rapid global spread of disease. A disease that spread rapidly from person to person could infect a significant fraction of the population before countermeasures could be devised.

A pessimistic, but realistic summary of the possibilities comes from the virologist Karl M. Johnson, who led the response to the first Ebola outbreak.

"So far we have been able to identify and deal with what has happened," he said. "But the great likelihood is that the whole globe may be suddenly exposed to something we can't deal with. You can't predict that will happen, but the odds get higher the more and more of us there are."

Joshua Lederberg, Nobel Prize winner and former president of Rockefeller University, warns that we will be hamstrung in dealing with future disease threats "if we do not come to grips with the realities of the place of our species in nature." We share a planet with animal and plant species that we carelessly destroy at will. At our peril, we ignore the relationship with trillions of microscopic life-forms with which we share our bodies and the globe.

BOOK

2

WHO LIVES LONGER?

CHAPTER SEVEN

RISE OF THE RISK FACTOR DISEASES

Excess weight. Elevated cholesterol. High blood pressure.

Almost everyone over age 40 now worries about at least one of these risk factors. More than 40 million adults are taking medication daily or are under a doctor's treatment to control these disorders. Many millions more are exercising or have changed their diet. The remaining fraction are unusually fortunate, just don't care, or promise themselves to do better tomorrow. The unspoken but underlying goal is to prevent premature death or improve life expectancy. These three risk-factor diseases have become the modern-day vehicle for translating this universal but vague aspiration into specific action.

The modern health-promotion apparatus has so effectively made the big three risk factors the centerpiece of healthy living that rare indeed are the individuals who have not heard the message. A strange partnership of citizens' groups and medical organizations, quietly bankrolled by food manufacturers and drug companies, has spent millions of dollars delivering the word to every family that reads a newspaper or watches television. In many medical practices, it is difficult to see the doctor without getting weighed and having one's blood pressure and cholesterol level checked. To many health-conscious adults, these three measurements define one's health status and longevity prospects.

Examined dispassionately, it is strange that they should occupy so central a position in the constellation of potential influences on health. Unlike most disorders, these have few symptoms to send the afflicted scurrying to the doctor for relief. In fact, cholesterol level and blood pressure can be determined only by medical testing, and naturally occurring changes usually cannot be detected by the individual. Severe obesity is painfully obvious to everyone, but for the majority who are overweight, the most identifiable symptom is mild discomfort and occasional embarrassment, particularly at times when little or no clothing is appropriate. These risk factor diseases not only are generally without symptoms, they are in themselves remarkably benign. They cause fatal or severe illness only in a tiny fraction of the most extreme cases. So how did such mild disorders become so important? It is believed they place one at increased risk for other diseases that are unmistakably fatal, most notably heart disease and stroke. And with obesity, a major danger is twice removed from a more conventional disease: it is a risk factor for high blood pressure, which is a risk factor for heart disease and stroke.

The rise of the risk factor diseases also marked a new stage in the relationship between doctor and patient, and between the medical system and society. Traditionally it required no expert to tell someone when he was sick—or healthy. When the patient decided he felt bad enough, he went to the doctor. This arrangement was not perfect. For example, millions of mild heart attacks were dismissed by the stoic as a case of stomach upset or an unimportant episode of chest discomfort. On the other extreme, doctors' waiting rooms were often filled with patients complaining of cold viruses or other uncomfortable but mild disorders for which the only remedy was rest. However, the arrangement was simple. The patient decided when he was sick enough to require medical help. Only then was the physician's expertise deployed to identify the cause of the patient's suffering and to provide whatever help was possible. No guarantee of a cure was asked or expected.

Cholesterol and blood pressure in particular were entirely different medical propositions. Now the medical system was taking the initiative, screening millions of people who were otherwise healthy, and telling them they had a disease requiring medical treatment. It is one kind of world when someone feels bad and asks a doctor for help. It is entirely another when the doctor tells an individual to spend thousands of dollars a year on a lifetime treatment program to curb a disorder that, to the patient, is entirely invisible. Few observers have appreciated the importance of this massive transfer of power from the individual to the medical system. Fewer still have realized the need to ask many more searching questions about this new class of medical treatments.

Given this new and sweeping power to define who is sick and who is healthy, it should be no surprise that truly enormous numbers of people have been found sick enough to require expensive programs of medical treatment. The National Heart, Lung, and Blood Institute—the arm of the National Institutes of Health responsible for heart disease research—defines borderline high cholesterol as any level over 200 milligrams per deciliter (mg/dl). Under this standard nearly two out of three adults require medical monitoring, and 38 percent require treatment. High blood pressure is also generously defined: 58 million adults require treatment. And the National Institutes of Health has similarly declared that anyone more than 20 percent over ideal weight requires a program of medical treatment, a sweeping definition of obesity that includes 35 million adults. For all the expense, energy and attention that medical treatment of risk factors has commanded, one would suppose the impact on life expectancy might be of a magnitude comparable with the extraordinary gains against infectious disease. Sadly, this is hardly the case.

Overall, the risk factor strategy for longevity has proved to be a terrible disappointment. It has consumed tremendous time, money and energy to produce remarkably few measurable effects on health or life expectancy. It has been marred by major scientific errors and treatment failures, and characterized by a style of massive medical overkill. Toxic side effects and escalating costs have been studiously ignored, and the benefits of treatment systematically exaggerated. Without question there are individuals who will reap great benefits from attention to risk factors. The great tragedy of the risk factor strategy is that the minority who may be helped are buried in a vast multitude numbering in the millions who will get no benefit; and many will be harmed unnecessarily.

This creates difficult problems for the inquiring consumer of treatments for risk factor diseases. However, one shortcut clarifies a subject in which there are otherwise no genuinely simple answers. Given just one question, ask, "What were the results of the treatment intervention, measured in objective experiments?" The reader will observe the surprising results of many such experiments in the pages to come.

The next four chapters will therefore focus on the strengths and weaknesses of the risk factor strategy for promoting health. What scientific evidence, what approach to longevity, and what kind of medical system brought these concerns to center stage? What are the likely benefits of controlling a risk factor? Separate chapters will address obesity, high blood pressure and cholesterol individually. All three, however, are part of a larger picture, components of a grand strategy for improving health in a era where the threat of infectious disease has reached an all-time low. Outlining these common elements is the central task for this chapter.

To set aside the health propaganda and ask hard questions about the results of the risk factor strategy is to enter a world that at first seems bizarre. Who would believe that physicians would prescribe an expensive and uncomfortable treatment that had a 90 percent chance of failure, and without knowing whether the 9 out of 10 failures would be harmed by the experience? Authorities continue to promote certain cardiovascular health recommendations after five carefully conducted scientific trials showed no benefits from this approach, and possibly harm. A government expert panel justified a massive treatment program for millions of Americans on the basis of a $120 million, seven-year clinical trial in which there were 38 cases of moderate to severe side effects for every individual who might have benefited.

Even a critical look at the actual risks is revealing. Consider this authoritative official report appearing in the *Journal of the American Medical Association,* and written by the federal Center for Prevention of Chronic Disease. It quoted the widely accepted and publicized estimates of annual heart disease deaths attributable to the major risk factors:

CORONARY HEART DISEASE

Risk Factor	Annual Attributable Deaths
High cholesterol	253,194
No regular exercise	205,254
Obesity	190,456
High blood pressure	171,121
Smoking	148,879
Diabetes	77,709

This is the usual scary fare fed to the public, generally without critical examination. But the following simple tally suggests just how far overboard the health promoters have gone.

The deaths blamed on risk factors for coronary heart disease total over one million. But only 500,000 *actually die* of coronary heart disease each year. That's just the start. These were risk factors associated with premature deaths from heart disease. But most heart disease deaths occur among the elderly. In fact, only 19 percent of the heart disease deaths occur in those under 65 years old. And only half of those deaths have been attributed to risk factors. The other premature deaths are blamed on genetic defects and other unknown causes. When totaled accurately, risk factors might account for 50,000 premature deaths from heart disease each year. These claims of a million heart disease deaths blamed on risk factors remain a gross exaggeration even if one assumes frequent double counting—for example, many of the obese would also engage in no regular exercise. It illustrates that one way to justify mass medical treatment is to exaggerate the risks.

To enter the world where risks are calculated and advice is created and tested is to begin a fascinating and instructive journey. A useful perspective requires an inquiry that ranges beyond the specific findings of scientific studies. There are great dividends from also understanding not only the mind-set of biomedical decision makers, but also the organizational structure that confines their thinking, on one hand, and gives it immense power over our lives, on the other.

The dramatic conquest of some infectious diseases, and the convenient disappearance of others, left the nation's system of doctors, hospitals and biomedical researchers in undisputed possession of the public's main hopes for a longer and healthier life. As we have seen, longevity is primarily a product of an orderly, enlightened and benign society, and the child of economic prosperity. But in the face of stunning victories over polio, and a new ability to tame terrifying killers like pneumonia and TB, it was the medical and public health establishment that emerged with the confidence, moral authority and money to pursue the perennial dream of a longer and healthier life. In the United States in particular, no time was lost and no expense was spared in constructing a system of truly awesome proportions.

In 1989 the United States spent more than $600 billion a year for health care, or more than $2,400 per person. This is more than the total income per person of countries like Brazil, Egypt or Mexico. The public supports 600,000 physicians at an average annual income of $120,000 each and pays the salaries of eight million other health workers. Health care employs five times as many people as are needed to grow our food, eight times as many as required to make our clothing, and eleven times as many as needed to build our homes.

The unmistakable style of American medicine is the aggressive intervention. When its aggressive skills are well matched to the problem at hand, modern medicine can be stunningly effective. Consider something as ordinary but potentially lethal as an inflamed appendix. In the year 1940 appendicitis was a leading cause of death for boys and girls aged 9 to 14 years, accounting for almost 8 percent of all deaths. Today half a million individuals of all ages undergo an appendectomy each year. The surgery is performed so safely, and the operation is so universally available, that in 1987 just 13 deaths from appendicitis occurred among young people in the entire United States, a seemingly pedestrian but nevertheless extraordinary achievement for medicine.

But when the can-do spirit of drastic intervention clashes with clinical reality, the results can be truly appalling. Faced with a fully metastasized cancer or irreversible damage to the heart, well-meaning physicians routinely sentence their patients to a miserable medically managed death, suffering through their last days sickened by radiation, incapacitated by toxic chemotherapy, or wracked with pain from futile open heart surgery. When the book *Final Exit* soared to the top of best-seller lists, medical professionals were greatly surprised and disturbed at the outpouring of interest in suicide as a kinder, gentler, nonmedical end to life.

The medical intervention approach also depends on a specific concept of health, illness and aging called the disease model. It is a deceptively familiar idea with far-reaching implications for questions of longevity. In its simplest iteration, it proposes that we are healthy, and presumably might live almost forever, unless afflicted by a disease, a specific disorder involving a particular system in the body. It might be an infectious disease such as cholera, influenza or pneumonia. It might be a chronic disease, for example, coronary heart disease, cancer or Alzheimer's, all of which involve complex degenerative processes. It might simply describe a group of people who deviate from the average on some biological measurement. For example, the National Heart, Lung, and Blood Institute once defined high cholesterol as the 25 percent of the adult population with the highest cholesterol levels.* So immense is the territory now spanned by the term *disease,* it can be conveniently defined simply as those disorders diagnosed and treated by doctors.

Once something is identified as a *disease,* a standardized approach and particular pattern of thinking define how it will be combated. Inherent in the concept of disease is the requirement for a medical treatment, even if it is not very effective. Success rates in the treatment of obesity, advanced cancers, and several major psychological disorders are discouragingly low. But this has little dampening effect because of the inherent medical mandate that any condition defined as a disease requires the response of treatment.

To define a condition as a disease is also an important social and moral statement. It places on society at least some of the responsibility—and possibly all of it—for devising, providing and perhaps paying for a treatment. However, to label an individual as diseased and requiring medical treatment also strips that person of freedom, independence and self-reliance. To be diagnosed with high blood pressure, for example, may affect income, life insurance and prospects for promotion. Particularly in law enforcement, but also in other occupations, the obsese can face disciplinary action for failing to lose weight. And at least one city government—Athens, Georgia—sought to reject applicants with high cholesterol levels, hoping to hold down insurance costs. But the intangible costs of labeling are more frequent and more important than direct job effects. No longer can the individual independently make the highly personalized daily tradeoffs that every individual does to maximize a perceived state of good health. Such people now require expert evaluation and management and are pressured to submit to the intervention, with a new set of health priorities imposed from the outside.

As the definitions of disease grow broader and more numerous, the freedom lost in this overall process can become significant. By age 65 a large majority of the population will have one of the three risk factor diseases, and many will have two of them. None of these millions have

---

*Because of technical mistakes, the program ended up targeting 38 percent of the adult population, and identifying 60 percent as requiring medical monitoring.

symptoms of ill health, except in a tiny minority of the most extreme cases. To escape prescribed medical treatment regimens for risk factor diseases may involve an even more all-encompassing self-imposed program of far-reaching changes in personal habits, diet and exercise. Marshall Becker of the University of Michigan School of Public Health describes this as "the tyranny of health promotion." He notes that those who fail to act against risk factors are often blamed if they subsequently become ill.

This extraordinarily broad use of the disease model to attack a variety of problems, ills and conditions may help explain a famous paradox pointed out by the Harvard psychiatrist Arthur Barsky. By objective measures such as life expectancy or being free of disability, the health status of the American public is notably better than 20 years ago. However, in systematic interviews, people increasingly say they don't feel well and are more worried than ever before about their health.

The past few decades have brought the absolute triumph of the disease model of health over an important competitor, the aging model. After World War II many physicians viewed coronary heart disease as a natural, inevitable deterioration of the circulatory system occurring with age. This approach has been replaced by the now prevailing view that it is a preventable disease. In the 1930s many physicians argued that high blood pressure was not a disease, but a natural and possibly beneficial adjustment to the decline with age in the kidney's ability to filter wastes out of the bloodstream. This viewpoint lost out because of evidence of excess deaths among those with higher blood pressure and the development of new tools to lower blood pressure.

The ascendancy of the disease model cannot be ascribed to an intellectual victory in a vigorous scientific debate; this was simply how activist doctors and health researchers thought about health problems, and they had won the assignment to improve life expectancy. It also expressed a politically appealing spirit of optimism. The aging model seems to bow to the inevitable, expressing to many an unacceptable fatalism. The disease model requires action and exudes optimism, suggesting a condition that can be prevented, treated and conceivably cured. Unfortunately neither model accurately describes the human species which, as it ages, becomes increasingly vulnerable to damage from many sources, including disease. It may be that for lack of a broader vision of human health, the assault on the risk factor diseases was doomed from the start.

The risk factor diseases are also the leading product of a particular approach to medical ignorance. With chronic degenerative diseases, biomedical scientists found themselves faced with processes of astonishing complexity. Blood pressure, for example, is the end result of interactions involving the constantly varying output of the heart, the expanding and contracting arteries, the amount of fluid retained in body tissues or removed by kidneys—all this regulated by cell membranes, arterial pressure sensors, signals from the brain and a cascade of the chemical messengers called hormones. But exactly why blood pressure often rises with advancing age is simply not known. Even larger zones of ignorance cloud scientific understanding of obesity and coronary heart disease. The men and women so deeply imbued with the intervention ethic of modern medicine were interested in finding the shortest route to effective action. So they embraced the scientific tool that had most quickly extracted practical results from the sea of ignorance. They turned to the science of epidemiology.

Epidemiology, as was seen earlier, is the systematic study of the occurrence of disease. In the pattern of who is afflicted and who is spared by disease are sometimes revealed vital clues to its nature. In the classic historical example described before, John Snow discovered that the households supplied by one London water company were 10 times more likely to get cholera than the customers of a competitor. This helped Snow deduce the microbial cause of cholera and the transmission route through water supplies before germ theory had been firmly established.

A more immediately relevant demonstration of the power of epidemiology occurred early in the twentieth century when the United States Public Health Service assigned an epidemiologist named Joseph Goldberger to investigate a mysterious disease sweeping through impoverished blacks in the South. The symptoms included severe weight loss, swollen and discolored skin blisters, and mental aberrations. The pattern of occurrence seemed to suggest a new infectious agent. Medical investigators had documented clusters of cases in numerous towns in rural

South Carolina, often affecting several members of the same household, frequently in neighborhoods with poor sanitation.

In the pivotal discovery, Goldberger studied an outbreak in a prison population. There he observed a critical difference between those who were stricken and those who were spared. The prison inmates and the prison guards and staff were in constant contact and drank the same water. But he found the disease occurred only among the inmates, never among the guards and staff. Had this been an infectious disease, he reasoned, it should have spread to at least some of the guards and staff. What was different was the diet. Therefore, he concluded, it must be a nutritional disorder.

To confirm his theory, he repeatedly inoculated himself and his wife with the blood and diseased tissue of recent victims. Neither Goldberger nor his spouse became ill. Subsequently he found out how to prevent the disease—through a nutritious and varied diet—but never learned specifically what caused the disorder. Today we know that the disease of pellagra is caused by a deficiency of the vitamin niacin. Among poor blacks in the South, it resulted from a subsistence diet of corn that was milled in a manner that destroyed the vitamin.

The achievements of John Snow and Joseph Goldberger suggested that in epidemiology medical science had a vehicle with a proven success record for venturing into the unknown and returning safely with life-extending ideas.

Today the findings of epidemiological studies have become regular fare for the health conscious with findings making national headlines every month. Does passive smoking cause lung cancer? Does fish oil reduce heart disease? What are cancer risks of eating red meat? Will vigorous exercise reduce the risk of a heart attack? Does coffee cause heart disease? Such studies, if published in reputable scientific or medical journals, are often reported without qualification or criticism, and are widely accepted as authoritative even when they contradict most previous research. It is unlikely that epidemiology would have produced such influential commandments for medical treatment, healthy living and eating were the severe limitations of the entire approach better understood.

Many an expert bows once respectfully to the most important logical failing of epidemiology, and then proceeds to ignore it ever after. All epidemiology can ever do is detect associations between events or traits that tend to occur together. It cannot by itself establish a causal relationship. Epidemiology is like a map to buried treasure: it can provide important directions where to look and where to dig. But what is found—or not found—can often come as a surprise.

Consider, for example, what happened in the early epidemiological detective work to identify the cause of AIDS. Two of the most important medical journals in the world, the *New England Journal of Medicine* and the British journal *The Lancet* published epidemiological studies showing the use of amyl nitrate "poppers" among gay men appeared to be the cause of AIDS symptoms; amyl nitrate use predicted the disease more accurately than the number of sexual partners. Learned studies were published suggesting how amyl nitrate—otherwise used to revive fainting victims—might cause the manifestation of AIDS that was then most frequently observed, Kaposi's hemorrhagic sarcoma, a rare form of cancer. (The reason for the spurious finding was that the AIDS virus spread initially among a particular social subculture where "poppers" were believed to enhance sexual pleasure.)

Other accidents are waiting to happen to the unwary consumer of epidemiological information. Particularly when one studies behavioral factors or biological measurements, certain traits tend to occur repeatedly together. For example, heavy coffee drinkers are also more likely to be smokers, to consume alcohol, be thinner and more tense. This has led to many spurious findings. For example, coffee was erroneously identified as an important risk factor for coronary heart disease. The underlying factor ultimately blamed was cigarette smoking; coffee drinkers were simply more likely to be smokers.

When studying diet, it is even more dangerous to try to isolate specific items. Not only do several foods tend to be eaten together, but also specific foods interact with each other and the enzymes in the digestive system depending on the form, preparation and other factors.

Under the best of circumstances, and when used with caution, epidemiology can be a powerful tool for uncovering new truths. Under almost all other conditions, it is a trap ready to mislead the unwary, and occasionally will snare even the most scrupulous researcher.

Consider Goldberger's bold attempt to confirm his theory about the nutritional cause of pellagra by inoculating himself and his wife with disease material. Fortunately they did not become ill. However, Goldberger would also not have become immediately ill had he encountered an infectious disease like chickenpox, mononucleosis or polio, in the days before vaccination. In these infectious diseases a large majority of the population acquired immunity at a very young age and, in the case of polio and mononucleosis, probably without even knowing it. His self-inoculation test also would have produced no immediate illness with a disease with a long latency period—for example, AIDS. What made Goldberger's conclusions convincing was an intervention study. The disease disappeared when the inmates were fed the same foods as the guards, and reappeared on a restricted diet. Unfortunately, the crucial second step—an intervention trial or other unimpeachable confirming evidence—was frequently omitted as epidemiological studies grew in popularity and influence.

Surgeon General Luther Terry's famed 1964 campaign against smoking was launched on surprisingly limited epidemiological evidence. The striking association between cigarette smoking and lung cancer found in men could not then be similarly demonstrated in women. And while tobacco smoke tar caused skin cancer in laboratory animals, it did not cause lung cancer. And no intervention study had demonstrated that quitting smoking provided health benefits.*

Because the later scientific evidence reinforced rather than undermined the initial finding, conventional wisdom held that the surgeon general's report demonstrated why science couldn't afford to wait for enough evidence to satisfy every skeptic. Protection of the public required immediate action on the best information available. It was, in fact, a very dangerous precedent. To fuse the aggressive spirit of American medicine with a remarkably low standard of scientific proof is an invitation for gross error. And as the next three chapters will show, such errors have occurred repeatedly and are rarely acknowledged or corrected.

---

*Later intervention trials also failed, mainly because of failure to induce participants to reduce their cigarette consumption substantially. Evidence of the health benefits of smoking cessation is based on less authoritative studies of former smokers.

CHAPTER EIGHT

OBESITY

It is an optimal state of the human condition to live in harmonic balance with the constant pull and tug of our numerous biological urges. They flood us with an unending chorus of requests for food, for air, for sex, for water, for exercise, for love and affection. To obtain fulfillment of those needs, our biological systems sometimes seduce us with the positive lure of sumptuous flavors and alluring odors. That failing, they turn nasty, sending forth obsessive thoughts that invade and dominate the conscious mind, or they turn loose gnawing hungers or feelings of panic. Because these demands sometimes clash, moderation has won the name of virtue over many centuries. But in many, a comfortable balance can be achieved most of the time.

In obesity, this harmony seems permanently disturbed. Apparently, something has gone wrong in the complex cascade of signals that get us unfailingly to the dining room table at dinnertime and up from our chair after consuming what we need and no more. In this seamless sequence of urges and action that regulates weight so efficiently for most people, a baffling malfunction has occurred.

The disorder called obesity—especially the milder manifestations—is widespread. Under the official but generous medical definitions used in the United States, 26 percent of the entire adult population is obese. There are major variations: 61 percent of middle-aged black women are obese, compared with just 12.7 percent of 20-year-old white males, and even fewer young black males, just 5.5 percent. And only about one quarter of the adult population is at so-called ideal weight—the level that actuarial studies show is associated with the longest life expectancy.

Although the data have been presented to the public in a much more alarming fashion, the loss in life expectancy for all but a small minority of the most obese could be measured in months, not years.

Obesity is also a harsh but revealing mirror reflecting a larger portrait of pitfalls of the modern pursuit of a longer and healthier life. Observing how a mild and mostly cosmetic disorder became a major risk factor disease requiring medical treatment for 1 out of 4 American adults provides an introduction to the problems of living in a culture of medical overkill. Thus, an examination of the risk factor disease of obesity is more than an account of a mysterious but generally mild biological disorder. Perhaps first and foremost it is the story of our medical and health system, how it operates, and where it fails.

While elevated cholesterol or blood pressure is an invisible problem to the patient, obesity is inherently a disorder that does spur individuals to seek help, but only in a tiny minority of the most extreme cases. It is primarily a cosmetic issue, and a vast service industry has grown up to meet the perceived needs. In the United States alone, dieting is reckoned a $30-billion-a-year business. It ranges from lavish health spas costing thousands of dollars a week to support groups gathering in church basements. Some of the biggest moneymakers, in the best tradition of American service-sector capitalism, are storefront franchises such as Jenny Craig, NutriSystem and Weight Watchers. Commercial diet companies quickly learned the same cynical lesson that the drug industry has converted into uncounted billions of dollars in profits: the most lucrative of all products are for conditions that are never cured and require a lifetime of repeated treatment—for example, lowering choles-terol or blood pressure, or losing weight. However, it is likely that no single factor caused the medical system to seek to seize the obesity problem from the commercial diet industry. The system was driven by the usual forces: the relentless appetite for more revenues, some scientific discoveries, and a particular pattern of thinking about risk and its reduc-tion. The outcome of the move to mass medical treatment for obesity was not quite so dramatic as the revolution brought by the cholesterol crusade and the war against high blood pressure. However, it is easier in the case of obesity to observe the basic forces at work—their strengths and their notable weaknesses.

While political issues are defined through debate and decided by vote, medicine is ruled by consensus and governed by guidelines. Little else, in a formal sense, controls the attitudes and practice patterns of the 150,000 physicians involved in primary care. A large majority are remarkably free to employ their independent medical judgment as they see fit. In fact, both the legal requirements of state licensure and the practical limits of what insurance companies will pay for allow much greater latitude than is exercised in actual practice, most of the time. But from the earliest medical training, the daunting complexity of their job has conditioned physicians to the necessity of applying a series of rules and guidelines.

To examine medicine from the inside is to realize the extent to which the physician's job boils down to applying an astonishingly lengthy series of memorized rules and guidelines. Those who seek to influence medical practice—whether a drug company or the national health authorities—long ago learned this. The starting point, therefore, for changing medical practice is the development of new guidelines representing a consensus of experts. That is one reason a consensus conference of specialists on obesity, held in 1985, would prove so influential in the rise of this risk factor disease. Another reason was the prestige and authority of the conference's sponsor—the National Institutes of Health, or NIH.

The NIH is arguably the single most powerful agency of the United States government in terms of influencing the health care the public will receive. It is not, however, immediately obvious why this is so. Its comparatively modest $8 billion budget goes almost entirely to finance and direct medical research. The NIH also has little power to tell anybody—except maybe grant recipients—what to do. The official mission of NIH is research, which is conducted mainly in medical schools. Its influence over what treatments are provided and paid for is simply enormous. A near-monopoly over funds for medical research provides the power to define what medical problems are going to be attacked, and therefore which issues will attract the attention of the most talented in the world of medical research. Most of the nation's leading experts on any particular medical subject head medical research units largely funded by NIH. These same experts serve on NIH panels, review grant applications from their colleagues, and are knitted together in an old-boy network of awesome power. Down in the trenches, the doctors who have to make treatments work for patients often do little more than apply and interpret guidelines. At the NIH, and among the coterie of experts that control each medical specialty, are found the powerful physicians who write the rules. This is true in cancer treatment, in cardiology and in the treatment of obesity.

Consensus is the unwritten rule of operation. Until a recent court decision, scientists who conducted NIH-sponsored research could not reveal or discuss their own findings without approval of NIH. Even senior researchers came to believe that if they dared to oppose NIH positions publicly, their grants might be canceled and their career left in ruins. While very few actual cases of such sanctions occurred, many senior medical researchers believe in this threat and therefore keep their criticisms to themselves. This is the invisible government of American medicine, presenting so monolithic a face to the outside world that few examine its actions. It is instructive to observe this organization and system in action on the problem of obesity.

The pivotal event that launched the medical treatment of obesity was a consensus conference, held in December 1985 at NIH headquarters in Bethesda, Maryland. Its NIH sponsorship meant any judgments would be widely quoted as authoritative interpretation of the best scientific evidence now available. The planning chairman was one of the leading figures in obesity research, Theodore B. Van Itallie of Columbia University medical school.

At this health summit, the central features of a new risk factor disease would be defined. The participants would barrel through 19 complex presentations in a mere one and a half days and issue an authoritative declaration. Critics of the NIH consensus process have long argued no group of thoughtful experts could conceivably assess such evidence on this breakneck schedule unless the outcome had been already determined in advance. However arrived at, the consensus conference on obesity took no position adverse to the interests of those who wanted to publicize, promote or profit from the medical treatment of the overweight.

The first and perhaps most far-reaching result of the conference was an unusually generous definition of the risk factor disease of obesity. It declared that 26 percent of the adult population was medically obese and required medical treatment. At current population levels that amounts to more than 40 million adults. To arrive at this figure the conferees simplified an existing but entirely arbitrary standard for being over-weight.

An earlier national health survey had arbitrarily defined the over-weight category as the heaviest 15 percent of individuals in their 20s. Since people typically gain weight with age, that amounted to 30 per-cent of all white males by age 50, and 37 percent of white women by age 65; and blacks tend to gain more weight than whites with increasing age. The conference adopted a second, simpler, rule of thumb that also had no independent medical justification: anyone more than 20 percent over the midpoint of the ideal weight range for each height was obese. The two definitions are roughly the same.

Such generous definitions offered great political benefits to the medi-cal system. Obesity researchers found themselves addressing a health problem of greater importance because it affected more people. Those interested in the potential profits from medical treatment now had a truly enormous market. Even the most selfless of health crusaders could conclude that with a more generous definition, more people could be helped with treatment. The individuals who would be harmed by this action were simply not represented at the conference. These were the millions upon millions of people who were just slightly overweight for their age who would now be told they were medically obese and required treatment.

The most detailed estimates of the actual health risks of being medi-cally overweight come from the life insurance industry, which has tabulated its mortality experience for more than 60 years. The most recent study, published in 1979 by the Society of Actuaries, reflects 28 years of industry experience covering more than 4 million individuals. These tabulations are the world's largest and likely most accurate source of data on height, weight and subsequent mortality. However, the mostly white and overwhelmingly male policyholders reflect only a narrow segment of a more varied total population. And except for noting already-impaired health, the study has no adjustments for other differences that also influence life expectancy. Nevertheless, the consensus conference panel and other analysts have turned to it as an authoritative major source.

The insurance data show that the longest life expectancy is observed at weights that are 5 to 15 percent below average—one reason that so-called ideal weights were set quite low. Death rates were elevated among those greatly underweight, and rose steadily again as individuals became increasingly overweight—a so-called J-shaped curve. The earlier in adult life the individual became overweight, the greater the risk of premature death.

The overall increased risk, however, is quite modest—especially among the majority of medically obese who are not greatly overweight. The insurance study also illustrates how actuarial arithmetic can be manipulated to provide a more or less exaggerated portrait of the same-level risk. Consider those 15 to 25 percent over *average* weight, a group roughly comparable with those 20 percent over *ideal* weight. In this group annual mortality rates were 17 percent higher than those of average weight. Among 1,000 such overweight men at age 45 there would be one extra death in one year's time. Over the next 25 years, the cumulative extra risk would amount to a loss in life expectancy of 3.6 months.★

For the minority of men who are greatly overweight—those 35 to 45 percent over average weight—the risks were still not exactly startling. For 45-year-old males, the death rate was 45 percent higher than for a similar group of average weight. This would account for two extra annual deaths among 1,000 men; over the next 25 years it would reduce life expectancy by 8 months.

For women—who would ultimately compose the majority of those treated for obesity—the risks were substantially lower. In the life insurance study, excess mortality was about one-half that of men of comparable obesity. In fact, a 45-year-old female who was 35 to 45 percent over average weight had no loss in life expectancy whatever in these data. Other large mortality studies, however, do show excess mortality among obese women, although the risks remain lower than for men. In the American Cancer Society study, for example, mortality risks for obese

★The insurance company calculations involve data for 25 years after the starting point, and are therefore incomplete. They should vary little from a true life expectancy calculation, which covers even the very oldest.

women are approximately 20 percent lower than for a similar group of men.

None of this should be interpreted as suggesting there are any health benefits from getting fat; the data are convincing that it is undesirable to gain weight. However, a balanced view suggests the mortality risks are quite modest. That is not, of course, how the consensus conference on obesity portrayed these same data.

"Body weight of 20 percent or more above desirable body weight constitutes an established health hazard," the conference statement said. "In extreme obesity the mortality ratio has been reported in a small series of being on the order of 1200 percent." To those who consider consensus conferences a medical insiders' game, it was no surprise that the statement incorporated the opening presentation of the conference organizer, Van Itallie.

In effect acknowledging the modest effects on life expectancy, he proclaimed that excess mortality was not the key issue. The real danger, he said, was that obesity was a risk factor for two other risk factors, high blood pressure and high cholesterol. In one frightening conceptual master stroke, Van Itallie had introduced an entirely new class of health hazard into the discussion: the risk factor for a risk factor. High blood pressure was found 2.9 times more frequently among the overweight, and high cholesterol 2.1 times more often. As terrifying as this might sound, the only way to understand the dangers of the novel and indirect idea of "a risk factor for a risk factor" is to return to the concrete bottom line. What is the effect on mortality? As the insurance data showed, the hazards are real but modest. All Van Itallie had devised was a more frightening way of expressing this.

Although the NIH consensus conference had defined a risk factor disease in which medical treatment for one quarter of the adult population was "strongly advised," it had intentionally sidestepped the most important issue of all: What medical treatments for obesity were available? What did they cost? Did they work? Without an effective way to help people lose weight and maintain the loss, a mass medical treatment program would be nothing more than an expensive exercise in futility and failure. And that, unfortunately, was the actual result.

Now that the consensus conference had helped define obesity as a national medical problem of major proportions, millions of dollars in potential profits awaited those who might offer a solution. It was time for an appearance by the third branch of the invisible government of medicine: the drug industry and other for-profit purveyors of medical equipment and products. Because these businesses seldom deal directly with the ultimate consumers, their central role in the operation of the medical system is frequently underestimated by outside observers. However, it is the drug and medical equipment companies that have the knowledge, money and organizational know-how to reach and influence the hundreds of thousands of independent medical practitioners. In marketing their products they spend an astounding $5,000 per physician every year—offering a dazzling array of information, trinkets, dinners, lavish conferences and other inducements. Their advertising dollars pay for the medical journals that provide up-to-date information; and rare is the medical conference held anywhere that is not supported by drug and equipment company money. Drug company money also cements together two other major players in the invisible government of medicine: the NIH and the medical school experts. The same medical school physicians who serve on NIH consensus and other panels also work as consultants to these drug companies, and are paid handsome fees to speak at the medical conferences that these companies finance. Finally the drug and medical equipment industry is the only other major source of funds for medical research units headed by the medical elite. It is a tightly interlocking system that would make apologists for the military-industrial complex blush.

For example, in late 1991 the NIH issued new guidelines for asthma treatment. A handsomely bound booklet was sent to thousands of physicians. On the back cover were the corporate logos of the drug companies whose products were recommended for treatment, and who paid for the booklet; inside were promotional letters from the drug industry. When it came to the selling of a new approach to weight loss, the interlocking system, with its inherent conflicts of interest, operated in a similar manner.

Sandoz, one of the world's pharmaceutical giants, was among those to grasp the potential new market for dieting as a medical treatment. Its subsidiary, Sandoz Nutrition, based in Minneapolis, Minnesota, marketed a medical diet treatment that fused two well-worn approaches to weight loss, combined in what seemed to be an innovative new way.

The first problem in the weight loss game is to get the weight off. Faced with even a minor deficit in caloric intake, the body mobilizes a formidable array of metabolic and other defenses to maintain its weight. As a result, even a strict, nutritionally balanced diet of 900 to 1,300 calories per day results in a weight loss averaging about one and a half pounds per week. And that average figure includes numerous periods in which the payoff for a week's faithful observance of diet is to weigh exactly the same as the week before. Under such circumstances a majority get discouraged that weeks of faithful deprivation produce such a modest result.

An alternative is to reduce food intake to levels seldom seen outside concentration camps—a true semistarvation diet of 450 calories a day. A Boston surgeon named George L. Blackburn had discovered that a very-low-calorie diet that included liquid protein would limit one of the most destructive of the body's responses to near starvation—it begins to devour its own muscle mass. Instead mostly body fat would be rapidly consumed. The approach had other advantages. After 48 hours, another body defense mechanism suppresses the hunger pangs. And because the diet consists of packets of flavored powder and water, the daily torture of tempting food choices also disappears. To those willing to tolerate it, this routinely produces 30- to 60-pound weight losses among the severely obese.

One critical drawback sank the liquid-protein diets when they first appeared in the 1970s: They could kill you. In fact, the FDA took over-the-counter products off the market after nearly 60 deaths had occurred. A sudden imbalance in salt and potassium in the bloodstream can lead to fatal disruptions in cardiac rhythm. In others, the body had still devoured enough of the heart muscle to weaken it fatally.

However, improvement in quality of the protein supplement minimized some of the dangers, especially to the heart muscle. And careful medical supervision helped control others. And while it might be difficult to arrange ongoing medical supervision in commercial diet programs, this requirement was perfect for a product that was going to be sold as a medical treatment. However, other major hazards of treatment remained, including dizziness, loss of hair, constipation, bad breath and gallstones. Given that the medical risks of obesity had been exaggerated, it became more acceptable to sell a medical treatment that also had its own negative effects on health.

The other approach to dieting, called behavior modification, traces its roots to the idea that obesity is primarily a psychological disorder. In this approach, individuals are taught how to count calories, order restaurant meals, and handle situations of unusual food temptation such as weddings. They attend weekly support group meetings and observe a strict, but nutritionally balanced diet. In the commercial sector this is the strategy used in programs such as Weight Watchers. While weight loss was slower, behavior modification had the better track record in solving the second major problem of dieting, weight regain.

It was a University of Pennsylvania obesity researcher named Thomas C. Wadden who tested the idea of a combined approach. In a widely quoted scientific paper, Wadden concluded that very-low-calorie diets produced the best immediate weight loss. Behavior modification performed best in sustaining any losses achieved. And combining the two approaches produced—at least after 18 months—the best result of all. To the optimists, and in obesity treatment there are many, it looked like a possible breakthrough solution to one of the most difficult of all medical problems to solve.

Of course, that is exactly how Sandoz would sell a very-low-calorie diet program called Optifast to the nation's hospitals—billing it as an innovative medical treatment, not as a way to slim down fast for swimsuit season. Sandoz was not alone. A smaller New Jersey firm, United Weight Control Centers, offered a similar hospital-based approach, as did a Boston-based company, HMR. And an entrepreneurial Maryland physician named William J. Vitale developed a program called Medifast that would be offered through doctors' offices. Medifast, Sandoz and HMR would, needless to say, cite the influential NIH consensus conference as establishing the medical need for a national treatment program. They also would repeatedly quote the conference's exaggerated portrait of the health hazards of being overweight.

Now all three critical elements in the making of a risk factor disease were in place: an authoritative government statement defining the alleged health hazards, what seemed to be a scientific treatment breakthrough, and the opportunity to make millions of dollars in profits. The semistarvation liquid-protein diet treatment was ready for takeoff.

By 1990 nearly one hospital in four had opened a diet center. Sandoz alone claimed that 600 hospitals offered its Optifast program, and HMR was not far behind, claiming 500 hospitals. Medifast said it had treated more than 560,000 patients through 16,000 participating physicians. The medical treatment through very-low-calorie liquid-protein diets had grown to half a billion dollars a year, according to Marketdata Enterprises, a market research firm. Compared with commercial diet centers, this was an expensive proposition—requiring an outlay of $1,000 to $3,000 for each patient. Because it was a medical treatment, however, the resources of the medical insurance industry were tapped for about half the total bill.

The Medifast program in particular pushed the practicing physician ever deeper into the dark gray ethical zone where medical judgment and potential profits intersect and inevitably conflict. For example, its brochure for potential physician participants provides, as is customary, selective citations from the scientific literature about the benefits of treatment. But it also includes an "Income Prospectus" purporting to show profits of $15,000 a month from an aggressive office program. And needless to say the Medifast program provides not only information about possible side effects but also ample supplies of waiting room brochures, promotion kits, plastic tote bags and fast shake jars. Would a physician who was aggressively developing a Medifast diet business examine this treatment as objectively as he would one from which he received little personal financial benefit? Would not a physician, whether consciously or subconsciously, inevitably discover increasing numbers of patients who might "benefit" from this treatment?

Hospitals proved no less hungry for new revenue sources. Faced with increasing pressures on hospitalization and surgery costs, these institutions diversified, opening wellness clinics, exercise facilities, diet centers and other health-related enterprises. "This was once considered a major growth area to diversify into," noted Steven Eastaugh, a professor of hospital finance at George Washington University. But would revenue-hungry hospitals ask hard questions about the efficacy of this program if it were popular and profitable?

Nevertheless, if the health hazards are genuine, and the treatment truly an effective route to better health, this strange partnership of government, medicine and private enterprise may not be a terrible arrangement. To run health systems entirely through cumbersome government bureaucracies certainly has little to recommend it. However, it is well known that hunger for profit has long tempted business to get careless with the truth. Less familiar but equally hazardous is the subtle but powerful pressure on doctors who prescribe a treatment to believe that it works—whether in fact it does or not. When medical optimism is joined in close partnership with the perennial hunger for profit, there is virtually nothing to protect the public from the resulting excess.

To witness a demonstration of that excess in action, consider what happened in 1990 when the major very-low-calorie diet companies appeared before a House of Representatives subcommittee that was inquiring into the activities of the diet industry. The prime focus was on abuses of some commercial providers and fly-by-night companies, but the diet-as-medical-treatment firms also had their chance at the witness table.

William Rush, the senior vice-president of Sandoz Nutrition, told the subcommittee how the Optifast program was different. "We do not treat cosmetic weight loss," Rush declared. "The average man or woman is a full 60 percent overweight." Taking a cue from the consensus conference, he added, "A full 40 percent of our patients are diabetic, hypertensive [have high blood pressure] or have high cholesterol, and as a result, will suffer from the even more life-threatening problem of coronary heart disease."

What Rush didn't mention, however, was that Sandoz had just launched a program specially targeted at those only 20 percent overweight—with possibly as few as 15 pounds to lose. (In a later interview, Rush conceded his testimony had been "inconsistent.") After the hearings ended, a Sandoz press release declared, "Marketers of the Optifast Program Receive Clean Bill of Health in Congressional Hearings."

In fact, this was not true. "The subcommittee didn't give anybody a clean bill of health," said its counsel, Graydon Forrer. "We're extremely concerned about advertising practices, safety and efficacy industry-wide."

The founder of the Medifast program, William J. Vitale, was little more accurate than Sandoz. He declared his company's program was "truly safe and effective."

A year later, the Federal Trade Commission charged both Medifast and Sandoz with making false and misleading statements about both safety and efficacy. While denying these charges, the companies agreed to tone down such unqualified claims.

Perhaps the most accurate testimony came from Lawrence Stifler, the head of HMR. However, Stifler, ever the diet crusader, spent most of his time showing the subcommittee five lean turkey sandwiches, and comparing them with a single calorie-laden pastrami sandwich with Russian dressing. Therefore, he had no time to address the disturbing medical study that showed 26 percent of patients on the HMR diet showed evidence of gallstone formation. (Asked later, Stifler conceded this was accurate but said he believed that later studies would show that most of the gallstones would resolve spontaneously and would not require surgery.)

One expects profit-making companies to put their products in the best light and sometimes overstate the facts. However, should one ask the medical experts for a more balanced view, it turns out that most are either consultants to the major companies, conducting research for these companies, presenting their results at conferences sponsored by these firms, or sometimes all three. For example, Blackburn, who did the early studies on liquid-protein diets, was a consultant to Sandoz. Van Itallie, who organized the NIH consensus conference on obesity, was a consultant to United Weight Control. And Thomas Wadden, who developed the combined approach to diet, worked for Sandoz. Presumably, all these and the numerous other medical experts with similar arrangements believe their independence of judgment is not compromised by such relationships. But hardly anybody stepped forward to publicize or even explain the critically important limitation of these very-low-calorie treatment programs: a majority gained all the weight back in the next few years.

This was not exactly how it was reported. For example, in May 1988, Sandoz invited 600 physicians and health professionals to a symposium on obesity. A Sandoz press release, describing one conference presentation, a scientific study using the Optifast diet, declared, "New research on very-low-calorie diets finds weight loss can be maintained."

It referred to a study of 400 members of a California health maintenance organization that was soon to be published in a scientific journal, *The American Journal of Public Health*. When the study actually appeared, it said: "There appeared to be little weight loss maintenance." This demonstrates the power of public relations in characterizing a medical study.

If one focused on the scientific literature, rather than pseudoscientific conferences sponsored by self-interested companies, the evidence was compelling that most patients regained most of the weight lost. The very-low-calorie diet had solved half the obesity problem—how to achieve rapid weight loss with manageable but real risks to health. However, even when combined with behavior modification therapy, it had achieved no measurable impact on the central problem of obesity: in a large majority, any weight lost was regained over the next few years.

One could observe a similar lack of long-term weight loss in the published studies of George Blackburn, the very-low-calorie diet promoter and Sandoz consultant. He wrote in *The American Journal of Public Health,* "The fact that only a minority of patients maintain long-term weight reduction should not be an excuse for therapeutic nihilism." Here Blackburn not only reveals that the diets don't work over the long term, but simultaneously illustrates the larger medical paradigm that diseases require treatment no matter how limited the actual results.

The gap between actual results and the promotional hype also troubled a Florida physician named Thomas J. Flynn, who was medical director of a hospital diet center offering Optifast.

"I am discouraged by the profit motive, the use of personality testimonials, the half-truths, the research results, and my own experience," he wrote in *The Journal of the American Medical Association.* He later conducted his own study of 255 consecutive patients in his hospital's Optifast program in Orange Park, Florida. After two years' time—a point that is still early in the cycle of weight regain—he found one-third had sustained some weight loss. But every one of his patients except four was obese according to the NIH definition.

"They come with dreams of wearing normal clothes and bathing suits again," Flynn said. "Those dreams are not accomplished." His results were typical of other long-term studies which showed that, regardless of the method used, from 85 to 95 percent regain all or most of the weight lost.

One could imagine the medical community exaggerating the hazards of a particular disorder provided an effective cure was available. For example, measles vaccination is a formidably effective and inexpensive treatment. So it is understandable why the one-tenth of one percent of children who might die of measles are highlighted rather than the 99.9 percent who would recover without harm. However, very-low-calorie diets are the opposite: both extremely expensive and ineffective. Also, in the face of dire peril to life, one can grasp the logic of offering the best treatment available even if the prospects for success are small. Patients with terminal illnesses frequently consent to—and sometimes demand— experimental treatments for which there is absolutely no evidence they might work. But to attack a generally mild disorder such as obesity with an expensive treatment that usually fails is the unmistakable sign of a medical system running uncontrollably to excess.

The immediate fate of the medical treatment of obesity hinged on something that separated it from practically all other medical therapies. In obesity, the effectiveness of treatment—or lack thereof—is simple to measure and immediately evident to the naked eye. It happened that one television performer—talk-show host Oprah Winfrey—came to sym- bolize both the apparent promise and the typical long-term result of the very-low-calorie diet. When the perennially overweight Winfrey ap- peared transformed into slenderness and modeling her size 10 Calvin Klein jeans, she created a national media sensation. She gave the Optifast diet all the credit. Her personal publicity blitz was so effective that Sandoz was deluged with more than 200,000 calls for information. The doctors, hospitals and providers who made up the very-low-calorie diet industry were ready and waiting, and in one year's time business nearly doubled.

Unfortunately, Winfrey's waistline became a kind of perverse barom- eter for industry prosperity. As she regained all the weight that she had lost, their business prospects plummeted. It was not that the fate of one individual—even a prominent media star—was so significant. But Winfrey was able to tap the sentiments of that enormous population of overweight individuals who desperately wanted to be thin. And her failure to maintain the loss was an equally compelling symbol of the typical experience.

By late 1991, at least 100 hospitals had dropped the Sandoz Optifast program, and company officers acknowledged that business was off 30 percent. Medifast said its volume was down by a similar margin. And HMR acknowledged that business was down 20 percent from the previous year. However, HMR's president, Lawrence Stifler, claimed that his competitors were vastly understating the real extent of the collapse. Overall, he said, the business had dropped by 60 percent. The Oprah Winfrey boom was a terrible mistake, he argued, because the real business of treating obesity is not achieving an initial weight loss, but setting up an effective program to maintain that weight loss. He predicted his company would survive because of its longstanding emphasis on maintenance. Others seemed ready to join the maintenance bandwagon. "Up until now, we have not concentrated on the maintenance efforts of these patients. We have concentrated on the weight reduction," said Medifast's Janna Thornton. "I can tell you that is going to change."

While the increased focus on maintaining the weight loss was healthy, the other response to failure was not. Given an approach that unmistakably failed the simple test of observation with the naked eye, obesity specialists simply changed the definition of success, employing medical jargon that could not be so easily challenged. Experts now began to talk of "medically significant benefits" of weight loss.

"Risk reduction constitutes a successful treatment program, not necessarily the loss of enormous amounts of weight," said Harvard's Blackburn, as quoted in a Sandoz press release. Sandoz director of medical affairs, Robert Hoerr, suggested that the obese would enjoy better health during the interval between the time when patients lost weight and when they regained it. Another emerging rule of thumb was that even a 10 percent weight loss was "medically significant." However, it seems self-evident that such modest changes cannot justify the expense and risk of a medically supervised period of semistarvation. More conventional approaches would suffice. And the life insurance studies had already demonstrated that any longevity benefits thus achieved could be measured in days or weeks.

. . .

Not only did physicians treating obesity find themselves prescribing a treatment with an 85 to 95 percent chance of failure; they had also unwittingly plunged hundreds of thousands of patients into a new zone of great medical uncertainty. What were the psychological and health consequences of subjecting the body to the stress of 16 weeks of semi-starvation and a rapid change in body composition—only to return to a point near where the patient started? Some would end up 5 or 10 percent lighter—the zone where "medically significant benefits" were now claimed. Others would weigh the same as when treatment began. And a substantial fraction would be even heavier. Would these patients be harmed by the experience? The handful of long-term follow-up studies focus so narrowly on trying to discover the secret of success that the costs of failure remain uncertain. However, there are substantial grounds for concern.

C. Wayne Callaway, a Washington, D.C., specialist in eating dis-orders, worries that periods of semistarvation may dispose individuals to binges of uncontrollable eating later on. That behavior, he notes, was observed among volunteers who participated in a World War II medical study of the effects of starvation. Such behavior was graphically por-trayed in a *New York Times* article by Molly O'Neill, who told of a lawyer who lost 143 pounds on such a diet. One day he hired a car and a driver and drew up a detailed travel schedule with 22 stops—all for food. In a seven-hour extravaganza he consumed 7,000 calories. In 13 days he regained 21 pounds.

Susan Wooley, a University of Cincinnati psychiatrist, is most con-cerned about the psychological costs of repeated failure—and the often scornful reaction of the medical professionals who participate in this failure. Treatment, she says, "may provide patients with failure experi-ences, expose them to professionals who hold them in low regard, cause them to see themselves as deviant and flawed, confuse their perceptions of hunger and satiety, and divert their attention away from other prob-lems."

The frequency and price of failure, however, should not blind one to the fact that every day, every month, some of the overweight do succeed in losing vast amounts of weight and maintaining those lower weights for long periods. The success stories not only reveal what strategies have the best chance of working, but also provide some tantalizing clues to the underlying nature of the problem.

Valerie Kirshy, age 49, has kept off 37 of the 45 pounds she lost on a very-low-calorie diet begun three years previously. Her name was provided by the Boston-based HMR as an example of a successful program graduate. A homemaker in the Boston suburb of Weston, she will tell you the answer is daily attention to maintenance, careful attention to the caloric content of everything she eats, and large amounts of exercise.

She walks 50 miles a week, burning off 100 calories an hour in the process. Her faithful program reflects the broader experience of weight loss experts who report that a willingness to exercise is the most important difference between those who succeed and those who do not. She also counts calories without fail—a task she says is almost second nature by now. Even after three years she still attends weekly maintenance meetings. When interviewed she was in fact trying to shed a few additional pounds. That morning she had breakfasted on a cup of vegetable soup. Lunch was a plain baked potato, two pieces of fruit, and more vegetable soup. For dinner, she will eat the family dinner of spaghetti with marinara sauce and a salad. The trick is to count out the calories and limit them to 11 per pound of body weight—plus any burned in exercise. "When I'm asked, 'Are you going to do this the rest of your life?' I say, 'I hope so.'"

"You trade obesity for a mild obsessive-compulsive disorder," notes Thomas Wadden. "You have to pay enormous attention to what you are eating." The big companies—HMR and Sandoz—also believe that their current participants will achieve better long-term results than the dismal performance reported in reputable scientific journals. They note that earlier very-low-calorie diet studies did not incorporate the long-term maintenance programs they now provide.

One hopes they will prove to be right. However, this sounds like a recurring theme in the frustrating problem of obesity treatments: There is always new hope, just around the corner. Meanwhile, millions of people are being told unnecessarily they have a dangerous disorder that requires medical treatment. In reality, most are merely overweight.

CHAPTER NINE

HIGH BLOOD PRESSURE

A bare-chested young man sat on a simple wood chair that had been backed into the corner of a featureless room. Strapped to his chest was a bundle of dynamite. Wires led to a huge alarm clock that could be heard loudly ticking away. A voice began to speak. "If you've got high blood pressure you're walking around with a time bomb ticking away inside of you ready to kill or cripple."

Millions saw this public service television advertisement. It was a memorable, dramatic centerpiece of the massive public health crusade to combat the granddaddy of all risk factor diseases—high blood pressure. From its initiation in the early 1970s, the campaign had important features that distinguished it from the more recent efforts to make obesity a risk factor disease. First and foremost, moderate high blood pressure constitutes a significant threat to health, and severe elevations place life in immediate peril. In this instance, not only was there a health problem; there was a solution. The discovery of a relatively safe means to lower blood pressure was a medical breakthrough of major proportions. The importance of blood pressure control has been sold to the public so effectively that today it is the leading reason for visiting the doctor.

In the case of high blood pressure, medical research probed beyond the simple and frequently misleading risk factor relationship found in epidemiological studies. Treatment was not justified solely on the basis of statistical associations that showed that stroke and heart attack occur more frequently among those with elevated blood pressure. In this case

elaborate intervention trials were held to establish—and to measure—
the actual effects of treatment on health and life expectancy.

The popularity and success of the war on high blood pressure made
it the model for the other two risk factor disease campaigns—elevated
cholesterol and obesity. Therefore, to examine the war on high blood
pressure is to be present at the very creation of this central medical
strategy for improving health and longevity. Many of the serious flaws
that would undermine the entire risk factor disease strategy may also be
observed. The U.S. health authorities, for example, in defining the
population that required medical treatment would include almost twice
as many people as under the Australian standard and five times as many
as under the British health guidelines. In the case of treating mild
elevations of blood pressure, overeager health policymakers got the
horse and the cart reversed. Long after millions of individuals had been
urged to undergo a lifetime regimen of drug treatment, a large clinical
trial was launched to find out whether this would be helpful or harmful.
When this and similar experiments were completed, it turned out that
the benefits were much less than expected, and the side effects more
widespread. The tremendous health benefits of treatment for a minority
were being buried in an avalanche of medical overkill.

It was also in the war on high blood pressure that the invisible
government of medicine learned how to operate effectively on a national scale. For example, consider the advertisement featuring the
young man with the sticks of dynamite. It was aired, free of charge, by
dozens of television stations as a public service. It was actually produced
by a group called Citizens for Treatment of High Blood Pressure. That
group's advisory panel included the physicians from the medical school
elite who had designed the blood pressure treatment program for the
National Heart, Lung, and Blood Institute. The money to make this and
similar advertisements was quietly provided by drug companies that
marketed high blood pressure medication. What a bargain for the drug
companies. They secretly financed the production of television advertisements run free of charge telling the public they may die unless they
keep taking their products! And when examined closely, the advertisements exaggerated the risks of high blood pressure for many people and
overstated the benefits of treatment. That is helpful if you're selling

drugs, but harmful if you're one of the millions who need to make an intelligent choice about whether to take high blood pressure medication. This chapter will examine those choices, and explain why they are so seldom presented fairly and objectively. The story of the war on high blood pressure, however, is also the story of a remarkable scientific breakthrough and the physician who played a key role in that discovery.

The handsome young physician on the medical service of Evans Memorial Hospital in Boston was in no condition to treat patients. Indeed, he was a patient himself. He had been brought from Los Angeles to see if the Boston University specialists who practice and teach at Evans Memorial might be able to help. His care became the responsibility of a 30-year-old physician named Edward D. Freis. The year was 1946.

As Freis examined the eyes of his patient with his ophthalmoscope, he did not like what he saw. On the inner back wall of the eyeball is a flat plate where optic nerves come together. When blood pressure rises far beyond normal limits, the valves that regulate the flow to the brain finally fail. Pressure rises alarmingly, and the brain tissues swell with fluid. This produces terrible headaches as the swollen brain presses against the rigid skull. Also, the pressure literally forces the tissues into the eyeball, which is what Freis noted.

Listening through a stethoscope, Freis heard bubbling noises in the lungs, a sound physicians call rales. Blood pressure can rise so high that the main pumping chamber of the heart, the left ventricle, begins to fail and can no longer fully empty its contents with each contraction. As a result, blood backs up in the vessels upstream, and in particular accumulates in the capillary network of the lungs. As this happens, the lungs fill with fluid squeezed through fragile membranes by the excess pressure. In severe cases like this, the patient feels a sensation of drowning when lying down.

The lab tests provided additional evidence of the patient's dire straits. His kidneys were also damaged and beginning to fail because excess pressure was rupturing the tiny valves that regulate the filtration pressure.

In the language of medicine, the patient had a condition called malignant hypertension. His blood pressure was almost double that expected in a normal adult of his age. In the year 1946 such cases were by no means rare. What made this case unusual was that Freis had a new research assignment: he was supposed to devise a new way to deal with the problem. This also marks a useful beginning point in the story of the direct medical assault on high blood pressure.

The first step in the long journey that would lead to an effective treatment had been taken more than two centuries earlier, in 1733. Stephen Hales, an English country clergyman of scientific inclination, tied a 14-year-old horse to the ground. He opened the femoral artery into a brass pipe, which then led to an enormously tall vertical glass tube. In the first known blood pressure measurement, he observed that the blood rose 8 feet 3 inches in the vertical column.

It was nearly a century before a French medical student, Jean Marie Poiseuille, made the first important practical improvement on Hales's scheme. He substituted a column of mercury, and noted that the same blood pressure that rose more than 8 feet in an open glass tube elevated the heavy mercury just about 3 inches or, in modern parlance, about 80 millimeters of mercury (80 mm Hg).

In 1896, an Italian physician named Riva-Rocci took the critical step that turned the measurement of arterial blood pressure into a splendidly simple procedure. Riva-Rocci fastened a cuff around the bicep and inflated it enough to collapse the brachial artery in the arm. Then as pressure in the cuff was allowed to fall, he observed the pressure at the exact instant that the blood flow resumed, which he detected as a resumption of the pulse at the wrist. It was now simple to determine blood pressure. This, however, measured only the blood pressure as the heart contracts, or systolic blood pressure.

In 1905 the Russian physician Nikolai Korotkoff disclosed that by listening to the same brachial artery with a stethoscope just at the instant that the cuff admitted blood again, blood pressure both at rest, diastolic, and during contraction, systolic, could be accurately measured. Korotkoff's method remains in use today.

To ensure that blood pressure remains within extremely narrow limits, the human body provides an impressive variety of interacting systems of both sophistication and beauty. The most elementary mechanism is to vary the output of the heart pump. Its output can vary from zero, for brief periods, to about 5 gallons a minute. The heart, moreover, does not dump its output into inert, hollow pipes. The diameter of the elastic blood vessels can be greatly increased or narrowed to maintain uniform pressure. To enable the arteries to respond to pressure changes, the smooth muscles in the blood vessel walls are held in a state of partial contraction at one-half their maximum diameter. Without the arterial capacity to make nearly instantaneous adjustments, the body would be unable to solve problems as elementary as getting out of bed in the morning without falling to the floor in a faint. As we stand up, gravity pulls large quantities of blood into the large vessels of the legs and arms. Blood drains rapidly from the brain, and without intervention, unconsciousness results. To balance these demands, blood vessels in the extremities can be narrowed to maintain adequate pressure and flow to the brain.

While these mechanisms deal with pressure emergencies, long-term regulation requires having the right total amount of fluid in the system. Not enough plasma and a heart will labor overtime to push blood through vessels that are narrowed to maintain pressure, and at the extremities supplies of oxygen and nutrients will be deficient. Too much volume raises the pressure and forces the fluid through delicate membranes to swell body tissues like a balloon and flood the lungs with fluid.

Not only must there be the optimal amount of fluid in circulation, it must contain the right amount of dissolved sodium and potassium. Most of the electrical impulses of the nervous system and muscles are transmitted through the movement of sodium ions, atoms with a positive charge because an electron has been removed in solution. Sodium ions are so critical that the concentration of dissolved salt in the blood plasma is not allowed to vary by more than 1 percent.

Maintaining the fluid and sodium balance is a principal function of the body's pressure filtration system, the kidneys. As the blood flow enters a kidney, most of the blood plasma is routed into a million tiny tubes called nephrons. As the filtrate flows through the nephrons, impurities are removed but most of the salt and water are returned to the blood. Any excess is excreted as urine. The chief wonder of this system is its versatility. It can reclaim more than 99 percent of the salt, or in a day's time excrete one-quarter of the total in circulation.

As soon as physicians were routinely measuring blood pressure they discovered numerous individuals in whom the resting-heart pressure was notably higher than the 70–80 mm Hg found in a normal young adult. Until this day, however, the cause of high blood pressure has eluded science. In most cases, no abnormalities can be found. In the language of medicine, with its unusual capacity to conceal ignorance and uncertainty, the condition was called "essential hypertension." In plain English, it means high blood pressure of unknown cause. And initially, it was also of unknown effects.

It was life insurance industry analysts, not doctors, who first perceived that elevated blood pressure might affect life expectancy. By the 1920s physicians were regularly measuring blood pressure, but had largely written off the occasionally elevated readings as a harmless by-product of aging, an adjustment to maintain effective filtration as the performance of the kidneys declined with old age. But the life insurance industry, with its central interest in how long its policyholders might live, concluded otherwise. By the late 1920s the actuaries had advanced the theory that people with high blood pressure die more quickly than those with average or low blood pressure.

With decades of systematic research now behind us, the evidence is clear and unmistakable. As blood pressure rises above a resting-heart or diastolic pressure of 80 mm Hg so do the chances of premature death, particularly from heart disease and stroke. (Diastolic or resting-heart pressure is the second and lower of the two numbers reported by medical convention, for example, 110/80.) There are no magic boundaries below which one is "safe," nor an identifiable point where the risks escalate dramatically. The most detailed figures still come from the insurance industry's Society of Actuaries, in a counterpart to its study of weight and obesity.

Among white males, when diastolic blood pressure rises from 80 mm Hg to the low 90s—what is today called mild high blood pressure—the mortality rate increases by more than 50 percent. When pressure exceeds 100 mm Hg, the chances of death are double those with average pressure. So-called "moderate" high blood pressure is usually defined to begin at 104 mm Hg. Furthermore, in developed countries blood pressure rises with age, and the younger the age at which elevated blood pressure is first observed, the greater the risk.

So how serious are these risks? A 45-year-old white male with mild high blood pressure—or a resting-heart, or diastolic, blood pressure of 92 mm Hg—has a risk of death that is 50 percent higher than someone with 80 mm Hg, the population average. In absolute terms this means that in a group of 1,000 men, we expect 5.5 deaths next year among those with high blood pressure, compared with 3.7 deaths among those who were average. Over a lifetime the extra risk amounts to just under two years of life expectancy—or about three times the health hazard of severe obesity. The risks for women are approximately half those of men—a pattern similar to obesity. Among blacks the risks are slightly higher; the more important racial difference is that elevated blood pressure occurs much more frequently among blacks, as does obesity.

All this information about risks, however, doesn't address the key question on which a reasonable choice about medical intervention might depend: how much of this excess risk can be reduced by treatment? As we shall see, it was in the benefits of treatment that unexpected findings occurred. The initial development of an effective treatment, however, depended heavily on the work of Edward Freis. In severe cases, his discoveries constituted nothing less than a medical miracle.

Freis had completed a residency in internal medicine at Boston University and wanted to make his mark in medical research. Aspiring research physicians usually seek a mentor under whose protective wing they may work while exploring some cutting edge in medicine. Freis found what he was looking for in the chief of medicine at Boston University, Charles W. Keefer.

Keefer had played a pivotal role in one of the most glorious of all medical triumphs, the discovery and mass production of penicillin. During World War II, Keefer had been the nation's penicillin czar, apportioning scarce supplies of what was without question the world's most important drug. One of Keefer's wartime colleagues was a physician named James Shannon, then head of E. R. Squibb & Sons' drug research operation. Shannon would become even better known as the first director of the National Institutes of Health. Shannon wanted to develop a drug to reduce blood pressure, and thought large doses of the malaria preventive pentaquine might work. Shannon turned to Keefer for help, and overnight, Freis became perhaps the nation's first specialist in blood-pressure-reducing drugs. Freis didn't choose his new frontier. It was chosen for him, by members of the elite club that rules medicine. The Los Angeles physician with malignant hypertension was one of Freis's first patients.

The patient had already been ruled out for the only competing treatment, the surgical severing of the nerves of the sympathetic nervous system. Deprived of the rhythmic signals from the sympathetic nerves, the smooth muscles of the arteries begin to relax, they enlarge in diameter, and blood pressure falls. It was a difficult operation, and the patient could look forward to a life of pain and debility. Its main virtue was that it seemed preferable to the alternative, which was death. But the surgeons at Boston University thought the young physician-patient was unlikely to survive surgery, and declined to operate. He thus was turned over to Freis, and quickly agreed to try the experimental drug, pentaquine.

The high dosages Freis gave him first seemed to make the patient even worse. He had terrible nausea and vomiting. He literally turned blue, because the drug increased the number of red blood cells that can't carry oxygen. He was in pain because the sympathetic nerves were affected by the drug. If he stood up too quickly, he was in danger of falling to the floor in a faint.

But his blood pressure went down. The fluid in his lungs disappeared. The swollen brain tissue returned to normal. He got well enough to walk out of the hospital and go home, although he survived only a few more months before succumbing to irreversible kidney damage.

To have seen such patients, says Freis, is to realize what a terrible problem malignant hypertension is and to appreciate that a drug to prevent it would be a godsend. Pentaquine, however, was abandoned as too toxic. It illustrates the fundamental balance problem of all such drugs: the trick is not simply to find a drug that will lower blood pressure, but to do so without doing more harm than good.

Freis's interest in high-blood-pressure drugs continued after he moved to Washington, D.C., to the Veterans Administration Medical Center. Soon, he heard rumors that Merck, the New Jersey–based pharmaceutical giant, had a new drug that might lower blood pressure. It was called chlorothiazide (or Diuril). He was able to get some of the earliest supplies available for investigational use, and quickly concluded that this time he had a real winner.

Chlorothiazide affected how the kidneys filtered the blood flowing through them, causing them to remove most of the sodium rather than returning it to circulation. The special brain sensors that monitor blood concentrations of sodium soon detected the loss, and triggered a series of events to compensate. The body increased the concentration of dissolved sodium by reducing the total amount of fluid, eliminating a quart or two in the urine. With less fluid in circulation, blood pressure dropped and, Freis believed, lives would be saved. It was one of an important class of drugs now called diuretics.

Freis was all set to a announce major high blood pressure treatment breakthrough at an American Heart Association scientific session in Chicago. His abstract was accepted, and the glory of a major discovery beckoned. But instead he was scooped. His old section chief at Boston University, Robert Wilkins, had also tested the new drug. Wilkins, a past president of the American Heart Association, didn't wait for the scientific session and the formal scientific approval it represents. He held a press conference immediately.

The incident illustrates another point that was true then, in 1954, as well as now. The research elite move from pharmaceutical companies, to major medical schools, the National Institutes of Health and the citizens' groups such as the American Heart Association. It wasn't even a game of musical chairs. It was a small group simply wearing different hats at different times.

Having discovered a relatively safe method to lower blood pressure created an unusual challenge for researchers like Edward Freis. Who else, besides the life-threatening malignant cases, might be helped by this wondrous new treatment? In medicine, most treatments do not resemble a business suit, neatly tailored to fit the subject. They help some people and may harm others. Many critical decisions in treatment involve distinguishing between these, and numerous failures can be traced to the failure to do so.

So where should treatment begin? At what point along the rising slope of resting-heart blood pressure that begins at 80 mm Hg, just about average, and becomes immediately life-threatening at about

130? The question would later become of pivotal importance in the war on high blood pressure because the numbers of people increase astronomically at lower elevations of blood pressure. The following table illustrates:

Diastolic Blood Pressure	Millions of People	Category
130	0.06	Malignant—life-threatening
115	0.9	Severe—damage imminent
105	1.0	Moderate—damage likely
95	19.5	Definite—increased risk
90	17.0	Mild—some increased risk

The implications were enormous. Was treatment appropriate only as a lifesaving intervention for the malignant cases, perhaps 60,000 people? At the other extreme, if it benefited the mild (or borderline) cases, here would be a drug for almost 30 percent of the adult population, an astonishing and medically unprecedented event.

Freis realized that was exactly the kind of question that could be answered with a medical intervention experiment called a randomized clinical trial. The idea is simple. A group of patients—in this case with similar elevations of blood pressure—are recruited. The subjects are randomly assigned to either the treatment group or a control group. Only the experiment's safety board knows which patients are getting the real drug and which are taking a harmless placebo. At the end of the trial, the differences in blood pressure, strokes, heart attacks, deaths and other events can be compared. Such experiments constitute the gold standard of medical evidence—objective trials in which both the risks and benefits of treatment can be systematically measured.

While simple in concept, Freis found that it took many months to evolve a workable design for a high blood pressure treatment trial. Then chief of medicine at the Veterans Administration Medical Center in Washington, D.C., Freis was able to recruit researchers at 14 other veterans hospitals to participate. When they started, the researchers were so strapped for cash that they had to hold their organizational meeting in the lobby of an Atlantic City hotel where they had gathered for an unrelated scientific meeting. The year was 1966.

The trial had been running less than two years when Freis first learned they might have a problem with complications. When an emergency tally was complete, he was appalled. There were already 29 adverse events, including 4 deaths. Three deaths came from the rupture of the largest blood vessel in the body, the aorta. There were also 5 nonfatal strokes and 2 heart attacks.

However, all the adverse events except 2 occurred in the control group among those with diastolic blood pressure of 115 mm Hg or more. This condition had proved greatly more hazardous than previously thought. The good news was that the blood-pressure-lowering medication appeared to have a valuable protective effect, a medical discovery so important the researchers halted the experiment to begin immediate treatment of the control group patients.

A report of the experiment was rushed into the *Journal of the American Medical Association,* whereafter almost nothing happened. There was little or no press coverage, and Freis detected little excitement in the medical community. People didn't know much about blood pressure and didn't worry. Nor were doctors much inclined to treat it.

Three years later, in 1970, Freis had completed the second phase of the clinical trial, among those with resting-heart blood pressures ranging from 90 to 114 mm Hg. Once again there were benefits of treatment, but they were not nearly so dramatic as among the patients with higher blood pressures. Furthermore, most of the benefits seemed to fall among the minority with the higher blood pressures, those with 104 mm Hg or more. The study, however, was necessarily limited by its modest size, a total of 380 patients, of which only half were treated. It could not reveal, for example, whether treatment reduced the single largest danger found in mild elevations of blood pressure—increased risk of heart attack. Stroke comprised a much smaller but still significant risk. The consensus was that the trials had unequivocally demonstrated benefits for the 2 million people with moderate or severe high blood pressure— leaving unresolved the potential harm or benefits for the 28 million with milder elevations. Limitations aside, it nonetheless was a contribution to medical knowledge of major importance, and once again, Freis was concerned that it would get no more attention than his previous study.

"This time I decided to get smart and have a press conference," recalled Freis. This yielded a brief wire service dispatch. And Freis still remembers getting exactly one sentence on Walter Cronkite's evening news in August of 1970. Given the landmark importance of Freis's two clinical trials, that did not seem like a great deal of attention paid to a vital health subject. But it was just enough to bring the matter to the attention of one of the most remarkable women in the history of American public health, Mary Lasker.

However, to understand the seminal role and contribution of Mary Lasker requires a brief look at the medical world she sought to influence, and ultimately changed. When Dwight Eisenhower warned of the dangers of a military-industrial complex in his 1960 farewell address, it would have been laughable to suggest parallel hazards existed in medicine. Throughout most of the twentieth century medicine looked like a chaotic cottage industry with thousands of independent, self-employed practitioners. Power in medicine tended to reside in the major medical centers, such as Boston University, Harvard, Johns Hopkins and Duke, where physicians were trained and new treatments developed and introduced. Traditionally the medical elite tended to behave like medieval barons, guarding their independence and prerogatives. As noted earlier, the major unifying force was the drug companies, which cultivated both practicing physicians and the academic elite with great care and lavish spending. Then medicine began to change rapidly. The first force that began to unify the fragmented centers of medical power was the billions of dollars in research grants available from the National Institutes of Health. The NIH did not rule medicine with an iron hand, but rather with the carrot of research money and a dizzying array of expert committees which tended to push the medical barons into consensus positions. When this new central edifice shared objectives with the increasingly large and powerful pharmaceutical industry, a combine was created, a health counterpart to the military-industrial complex. And like the military, it could tap a nearly inexhaustible wellspring of public concern, which invested health with the same passionate importance as national security.

By the year 1970, the NIH was already enormous, but in many ways a sleeping giant, its potential power partly limited by an ivory tower commitment to pure research. This was one policy that Mary Lasker was determined to change. How one wealthy, stylish and energetic widow could hope to accomplish changes on such a scale is an object lesson in how the nation's capital works.

Mary Lasker was already a successful businesswoman and health activist when she married Albert, a millionaire New York advertising man, a founder of the firm that ultimately became the advertising giant Foote, Cone, and Belding. The Laskers established a foundation bearing their name, and Mary would mount one of the most formidable political operations in the world of health and medicine. After Albert Lasker died of cancer in 1954, she continued her health crusade with renewed vigor.

She could do it all. She knew how to reach and mobilize the public. She had revitalized the American Cancer Society, changing it from a small and sleepy group to an active citizens' lobby. Her Washington operatives covered Capitol Hill with a thoroughness that would impress any defense contractor fighting to save an embattled weapons system. She built a national network of important academic physicians, such as Michael DeBakey, J. Willis Hurst and Paul Dudley White, and orchestrated their appearances at congressional hearings. And she worked right at the top. She was a friend of Bess Truman, an early supporter of John F. Kennedy, and she planted trees with Lady Bird Johnson. This dazzling array of skills was focused on a single purpose: promoting medical research and treatment.

She was the driving force behind President Nixon's massive war on cancer, a still controversial redirection of the National Cancer Institute from basic research to promoting new treatments for immediate clinical use. Mary Lasker was no less interested in diseases of the circulatory system. She was instrumental in the creation of the National Heart, Lung, and Blood Institute and served on its first advisory panel. It would be hard to find anyone who played a larger role in knitting together the pieces of the biomedical research establishment and making it a formidable national force.

When Mary Lasker read Edward Freis's landmark blood pressure trials, she decided that something had to be done. As was her habit, she went straight to the top, to her friend, Elliot Richardson.

Richardson still recalls the day she showed up in his office, bearing copies of Edward Freis's two clinical trials. Richardson was then secretary of Health, Education and Welfare in the Nixon administration.

"I remember thinking, 'Jesus Christ, this is serious. Something has to be done,' " he said. Outsiders were later to believe another event might have influenced the intensity of his interest. His father had been chairman of the surgery department at Harvard and had been incapacitated by a stroke at age 50. Richardson picked up the telephone and called Theodore Cooper, who then headed the National Heart, Lung, and Blood Institute. (Today he heads Upjohn, a major pharmaceutical company.)

Cooper and Richardson met the next day to plan a national campaign to educate the public and the medical profession about the benefits of treatment. The nation's war on high blood pressure had been officially launched. Whether measured in millions of prescriptions, billions of dollars, or lives affected, the results must have outstripped their wildest dreams.

In the zeal to help, little attention was paid to the unfortunate fact that the most important questions about mass treatment of high blood pressure had not yet been answered. This problem was eloquently described by Charles C. Edwards, then commissioner of the Food and Drug Administration.

"We all recognize there are some very difficult unanswered questions about hypertension," Edwards told a conference that Cooper held to kick off the national effort. "A quick look at the medical literature reveals disagreement on what constitutes true hypertension, on the reliability of routine screening techniques and also on the indications for treatment of the disease." In short they didn't know who had the disease, who would benefit or if they could accurately locate those at risk. Edwards, however, quickly concluded, that was "no excuse for inactivity." He portrayed the predominant style of American medicine: act immediately and aggressively. Worry about the skeptics and the details later.

In only a few years' time the nation's attitude toward high blood pressure was transformed. Spearheading the media drive to change public attitudes was a group called Citizens for Treatment of High Blood Pressure, headed by Mike Gorman, a savvy former Washington newspaperman and longtime Lasker lobbyist. The newspapers and the airwaves were flooded with messages about the dangers of "the silent killer." Eppie Lederer lent her powerful voice and influential "Ann Landers" column to the cause. Civic groups and businesses launched mass screening programs.

The drug companies plunged ahead with energy and enthusiasm to "educate" physicians about what proved to be the largest market for prescription drugs in the nation's history. They sponsored weekend getaways for physicians and their wives, special symposiums at luxury resorts. They beat on the doors of doctors' offices from coast to coast.

Often it was hard to tell the players apart. As noted earlier, public service advertisements were produced by Citizens for Treatment of High Blood Pressure, which was headed by Mary Lasker and run by Gorman. However, the production costs were paid by drug companies selling high blood pressure medication, especially Merck (chlorothiazide) and occasionally CIBA-Geigy (reserpine). Was this a laudable public service warranting free television time or a shrewd marketing scheme for the drug industry that concealed their role? It was probably both.

In another operation, the Lasker group persuaded Congress to earmark funds for state and local high school blood pressure education programs. Gerald Wilson, the current director of Citizens for Treatment of High Blood Pressure, estimates the legislation spawned 2,000 to 3,000 such programs. The 5-inch-thick community guide had the government's blessing and featured an introductory message from Edward I. Levy, who succeeded Cooper as head of the National Heart, Lung, and Blood Institute. (Levy later became the head of the research subsidiary of Sandoz.) However, the manual was written, published and paid for by Merck, which also offered physicians its own line of informational pamphlets.

It was a remarkable transformation of Edward Freis's pioneering work. Starting from a medical journal article that hardly anyone had read, the treatment of high blood pressure would generate more visits to the doctor than almost any other medical condition. A huge majority of all Americans now know their blood pressure is important. What had occurred was epochal in American medicine. It was in part a massive public health crusade. It could also be described as the medical establishment introducing a major new product line—treatment for high blood pressure. And it also marked the coming of age of the nation's medical-industrial complex, the textbook case of how the drug companies, the government and the medical community could operate effectively together.

For his efforts in launching the war on high blood pressure, Elliot Richardson was given one of the nation's most prestigious awards in medicine. Named for the sponsoring foundation, it is called the Lasker Award. At a ceremony to receive the award, Richardson sat at the head table with Mary Lasker, and he joked a little with her.

"You should have given it to yourself," he said.

In a nation less inclined to rush the blessings of medical treatment to the multitudes, some hard questions might have been asked at the outset. Freis's clinical trials proved to almost everyone's satisfaction that treatment worked at moderate and severe elevations of blood pressure, especially to prevent direct physical damage to the eyes, heart and kidneys. But that covered only about 1 in 20 people classified as having "high blood pressure." In this group the benefits were unquestioned. Were treatment limited to this group, high blood pressure would have become a medical problem in the league with diabetes or thyroid disorders, important but far from the silent killer threatening millions of American adults.

High blood pressure got its menacing reputation from its assumed role in heart disease. For every death directly resulting from hypertension, the condition was implicated by statistical association in 22 deaths from coronary heart disease, and another 6 from stroke. And here the dangers weren't limited primarily to the small minority with severely elevated blood pressures. Even among persons with mild high blood pressure, from 90 to 104 mm Hg, the risk of heart attack was double that of persons with normal pressure, and as blood pressure increased, so did the risk.

If those with high blood pressure are more likely to suffer a heart attack, can there be any doubt that lowering it with medical treatment will also reduce the danger? In the language of epidemiology, elevated blood pressure was ranked an important risk factor for coronary heart disease. Furthermore, while no causal relationship had been proved, it certainly was plausible that higher pressures would exacerbate any problems caused by the degenerative process occurring in the arteries. But some researchers were not so sure. Elevated blood pressure was the effect of some other disorder, they argued, and simply changing the blood pressure was pointless without getting at the underlying cause. The analogy is the rise in body temperature in response to infection. Lowering the body temperature does not kill microbial invaders. Reducing blood pressure would work no better, they argued.

Thus, to assume that reducing a risk factor such as high blood pressure will also prevent heart attacks or stroke required a leap of blind optimism. The more cautious would insist on a carefully controlled clinical trial to find out the truth, but that would entail many additional years of research. In a manner unique to the American style of medicine, the United States tried both approaches.

At the same time high blood pressure treatment was being aggressively promoted to millions of Americans, plans were made to conduct a scientific experiment to find out whether such treatment was justified. The result was a massive clinical trial called the Hypertension Detection and Follow-up Program, or HDFP. Physicians in Britain and Australia opted for a more cautious strategy: before promoting mass treatment of mild high blood pressure they wanted to find out the benefits. They too launched large clinical trials. All three efforts were targeted, not at the minority with severe high blood pressure—where Freis's evidence was accepted—but at the millions with mild elevations. The results were finally available several years later, and they surprised everyone.

It became unequivocally clear that high blood pressure treatment had little or no effect on the prime killer, coronary heart disease, which accounts for 8 out of 10 deaths associated with elevated blood pressure. None of the three large trials—United States, British and Australian—showed a measurable effect. Worse yet, there is fragmentary evidence that under some circumstances aggressive blood pressure treatment may contribute to heart attacks rather than prevent them, especially if combined with a simultaneous effort to reduce cholesterol. In an unrelated experiment, the National Heart, Lung, and Blood Institute reported that treating high blood pressure among those with slight irregularities in the electrical activity of the heart might cause, rather than prevent, fatal heart attacks. Other studies suggested that lowering blood pressure too aggressively, more than about 10 mm Hg, also might cause heart attacks. Finally, some blood pressure medication appeared to raise blood cholesterol levels, which would increase another risk factor for heart disease.

Although the threat of a premature heart attack was used to justify treatment to millions of Americans, little was said when it became clear the treatment didn't reduce this risk. The health authorities were saved from a major fiasco when the trials did show one important benefit— even among mild cases of high blood pressure.

Even at modest elevations of blood pressure, treatment proved dramatically effective against strokes, both fatal and nonfatal. In all three trials the incidence of stroke was reduced by 30 to 40 percent. To reduce the incidence of this frequently deadly and often debilitating event is still an important achievement in chronic disease prevention. But there was no immediate explanation why treatment should have so little effect on heart attacks and work so well against stroke, especially when heart attacks and many strokes appear to be the result of the same disease process.

Given that blood pressure drugs have grown to become the most frequently prescribed class of drugs, it is revealing to examine directly the actual results of the largest, most recent and best-designed clinical trial. The British studied the health status of 17,354 men and women with diastolic blood pressure ranging from 90 mm Hg to 104 mm Hg. The participants were prescribed daily medication for five years. However, one half received the drug, the other half an identical-looking but harmless placebo. These are the results:

	Treatment Group	Placebo Group	Difference
Subjects	8,700	8,654	
Strokes	60	109	45%
Coronary events	222	234	Not significant
Deaths—all causes	248	253	Not significant

The striking result is the beneficial effect of treatment on stroke. Of the three risk factor diseases, blood pressure is the most important, and this is the greatest effect yet established for a major risk factor intervention. However, the other differences are so small that they could easily have occurred by chance, and are not statistically significant. The table also provides an overall perspective and balance that are omitted from promotional material used to sell treatment to the public. It is true—as the public has been told repeatedly—that treating even mild elevations of high blood pressure dramatically reduces the risk of stroke. However, restating the same results in other language, it can also be said that the trial shows that if 1,700 persons were treated for one year, 1,699 will get no benefit. The medical axiom that prevention is always better than treatment remains open to question when the actual benefits are so small.

The British and the Australians also discovered an unexpected benefit of forgoing treatment. Almost half the untreated group got better anyway. In the British trial, blood pressure in 40 percent of the untreated controls declined below 90 mm Hg without intervention. In the Australian trial 47 percent of the control group fell below the threshold for treatment. This meant that many of those taking medication could reduce the dosage and ultimately do without it.

However, ceasing medication without systematic monitoring by a physician can be hazardous, because in some cases blood pressure begins to rise steadily and can reach levels that are dangerous under any reasonable treatment standard.

Although the British trial showed no effect on mortality, when all the trials were analyzed together it is theoretically possible to search for effects too small to be apparent in even a single large experiment. This kind of analysis suggests that treatment prolongs life very slightly, perhaps an 11 percent reduction in risk. Among all the risk factor diseases, high blood pressure treatment is alone in showing even a small effect on life expectancy. This means, for example, that someone with mild high blood pressure could reduce the excess risk of dying from 50 percent to 44.5 percent. Put another way, treating 1,250 people at this level of risk for one year might save one life. Because treatment had little or no effect on heart attacks, and prevented only some of the strokes, that leaves almost 90 percent of the risks of high blood pressure remaining despite treatment.

The life-prolonging benefits, however, are spread unevenly among different kinds of participants. The largest benefits went to black women, who suffer unusually high rates of high blood pressure and stroke. The smallest benefits—and possibly net harm—were found among white women. Among all women in the British trial and the white women in the U.S. effort, more deaths occurred among those treated than those not treated. These potentially harmful effects received little attention and analysis. In the U.S. study the finding was simply dismissed: "Any inference that white women should not be treated is unjustified."

Others were not so sure. Consider the actual data from the British trial, this time separated by sex:

TOTAL DEATHS

	Treatment	Control
Women	91	72
Men	157	181

The larger number of deaths among the women treated for high blood pressure differences hover on the borderline of statistical significance, and might have occurred by chance. Therefore, it cannot be said that treatment was proved harmful to women, even though deaths were more frequent among those treated. The trial does prove that treatment was less beneficial to women than to men. It remains possible, but not proven, that blood pressure treatment increases mortality in women.

"It ought to be of great concern in the United States that today women with mild high blood pressure are treated in greater numbers than men," said Rodney Jackson, a New Zealand cardiovascular specialist who studied the United States' high blood pressure program. "It is quite possible this treatment achieves more harm than good."

Today 46 percent more women than men in the United States are treated for high blood pressure.

Many people might nevertheless be satisfied with a lifelong drug treatment that offered substantial protection against stroke, and perhaps a small chance it might save their lives. This might be advertisement enough except that such medical treatment must inevitably cause harm as well as benefit—especially an intervention into one of the most essential and central mechanisms of the human body. Since the days of the ancient Greeks, when Panacea was enthroned as a daughter of the god of medicine, mankind has wanted magical cures without risk. With treatment of high blood pressure we got something else indeed.

The most important harm caused by the mass treatment of high blood pressure may be the most difficult to document. Call it the reverse placebo effect. The powerful effects of the placebo have been extensively documented. Some patients with an optimistic outlook get better even when the therapy is known to be ineffective or even an outright sham, with the physician only pretending to provide it. At the extreme, writers such as Norman Cousins (Head First: the Biology of Hope) and Bernard Siegel (Love, Medicine and Miracles) have widely publicized what seem to be remarkable responses to little or no treatment other than large amounts of optimism and a powerful will to live.

The reverse placebo effect begins when medical experts seek out millions of otherwise healthy people without symptoms of ill health and tell them they have a dangerous disease, high blood pressure, that requires immediate and continuing medical treatment. Some theorists, such as health iconoclast Ivan Illich, argue that the act of telling people they are sick makes them ill because it takes without consent the essence of health and vitality, namely being independent and in control of one's own destiny. Not only does an outside expert find that your health is in danger, this expert asserts that only he can keep you safe.

In medical terms, it is called labeling, and it does not affect everyone uniformly any more than does its opposite number, the placebo. (Some people are delighted to be taken care of and welcome outside direction.) But it was in the treatment of high blood pressure that the negative effects of labeling were most clearly identified and objectively measured. One of the earliest warnings came from pollster Lou Harris, who reported in 1973 that people who had been told they had high blood pressure reported missing twice as many days of work due to illness as those with normal blood pressure or those who had high blood pressure but didn't know it. Even better-controlled studies confirmed the findings.

"When you tell people they are sick, people begin to behave as if they are ill," said Marshall Becker, associate dean of the University of Michigan School of Public Health and a leading scholar on health behavior. As noted earlier, the label of high blood pressure can also have more direct adverse effects: loss of promotion, early retirement, higher insurance costs.

In extreme cases, the diagnosis of high blood pressure alone can cause great harm. "The fear of catastrophic illness or disability that can follow the identification of hypertension may be so overwhelming as to be incapacitating," noted medical consultant Campbell Moses in a presentation to a symposium at the New York Academy of Sciences. This is the dark opposite of the miracle cures attributed to positive mental attitudes.

Unfortunately, the adverse consequences of treatment are not limited to what goes on inside people's heads. There are also direct physical ill effects. When the war on high blood pressure was launched, the magnitude of the problem could not have been predicted by the two Veterans Administration trials, which reported only 2 cases of apparent drug toxicity among 380 patients. Also, the intervening years brought a wide variety of new drugs onto the market. Competing drug companies developed other diuretics, which blocked the retention of salt, and other compounds which worked entirely differently. Beta blockers caused the blood vessels to enlarge by inhibiting the signals sent down the sympathetic nervous system. ACE inhibitors neutralize hormones that can cause blood vessels to contract. There would be many more drugs, but larger and longer trials would also paint a much less favorable treatment picture.

In the Hypertension Detection and Follow-up Program, 33 percent of participants had to be withdrawn from drug treatment because of definite or probable drug side effects. In the British Medical Research Council trial, 19 percent were withdrawn. In the Australian trial 38 percent withdrew (however, that figure includes individuals who quit for other reasons). In Britain, where reported complications were fewest, researchers said they suspected their figures "were probably lower than the true incidence since not all reactions will have been mentioned by patients." (However, the reported benefits in each trial were unquestionably diluted because those who didn't tolerate the drugs were nevertheless classified as "treated."*)

---

*Inability to tolerate a drug because of side effects is as serious a limitation to treatment as failure to reduce the targeted adverse events.

The most frequent side effects were impotence in men and fatigue, lethargy or depression in both sexes. Of perhaps greater medical significance but slightly less frequent occurrence were gout and mild diabetes, called impaired glucose tolerance. The figures vary from study to study, but are substantial. About 10 percent of men reported impotence or sexual dysfunction, and 10 percent of both sexes reported weakness, lethargy or drowsiness. There were important differences by drugs. The diuretics, such as chlorothiazide, caused gout and mild diabetes more frequently. Both diuretics and beta blockers caused lethargy, shortness of breath and headache. Reserpine, used in cases where blood pressure is unusually resistant to change, frequently can cause depression.

Overall, the ratio of side effects to benefits is not favorable. In the British trial, for example, there were 14 cases of impotence, gout or mild diabetes for every stroke prevented.

A debate continues in medicine about whether the clinical trials overstate or understate the incidence of side effects. The optimists say side effects in normal medical practice occur less often because practicing physicians can switch drugs, tailor doses, and make other adjustments that can't be allowed in a rigidly controlled clinical trial. Pessimists note that the clinical trials used carefully selected, highly motivated volunteers who were treated without cost under ideal circumstances. In regular medical practice, they argue, too many physicians lack the training and fail to commit the time to fine-tune high blood pressure treatment. There appears to be substantial truth in both positions. It is also likely that many of those who experience side effects elect not to continue the medication.

The frequent adverse effects raise the question of how many patients with mild hypertension would elect treatment if candidly briefed on the risks and benefits. Here Campbell Moses speaks eloquently of the physician's dilemma:

"Obviously, when somebody in the near future has to try to communicate these possible adverse effects to patients . . . this will be a task requiring the wisdom of a Solomon and the communications ability of a Shakespeare if we are to achieve compliance without paralyzing fear."

How do risks and benefits compare for treatment of mild high blood pressure? A simple and objective summary came from the British Medical Research Council:

"The trial has shown that if 850 mildly hypertensive patients are given active antihypertensive drugs for one year, about one stroke will be prevented. This is an important but infrequent benefit. Its achievement subjected a substantial percentage of the patients to chronic side effects, mostly but not all minor."

This assessment, however, omits the life-prolonging effects of treatment (because no such benefits were detected in the British trial). The life-prolonging effects are small enough, though, that even modest numbers of adverse effects can tip the scales against treatment. One theoretical analysis, for example, found the lifesaving benefits of treatment worthwhile unless treatment degraded the quality of life. If treatment reduced the quality of life by just 2 percent on the average, the harm would outweigh the benefits, the study concluded. Given the high frequency of moderate side effects in blood pressure treatment, it is likely that treatment reduces the quality of life by at least this small amount.

Such studies illustrate why the massive medical assault on this risk factor produced so little effect on health status and longevity of the public. A partnership of overzealous health authorities and profit-hungry drug companies extended a genuinely beneficial treatment into large population groups where the benefits were equivocal at best and inevitably harmful to some. Among those leading the American medical establishment, almost nobody acted to protect the public from the very real danger of getting entirely too much of a good thing.

CHAPTER TEN

CHOLESTEROL

In September 1991, the world's second-largest medical publication, the *Journal of the American Medical Association,* published the long-term follow-up of an important clinical trial with 1,222 subjects. In the kind of experiment that constitutes the most convincing of medical evidence, researchers in Finland had simultaneously reduced the two most important risk factors for coronary heart disease, elevated cholesterol and high blood pressure.

The investigators had to overcome important obstacles that had doomed several other such trials to failure. Cholesterol levels in particular have proved difficult to lower over the long term, and several expensive efforts to demonstrate health benefits have failed because no meaningful change was achieved. In this trial, however, the investigators lowered cholesterol and blood pressure enough to report a 46 percent combined risk factor reduction in 612 middle-aged businessmen. (Another 610 otherwise similar subjects were not treated and served as the control group.) Disappointing results in earlier trials had also led many investigators to believe that it would take many years—perhaps a decade or more—to realize the full benefits of the intervention. In this instance treatment had continued for five years, and the benefits were monitored for an additional decade. Finally, previous studies had not demonstrated an effect on the number of lives saved or lost; small but tantalizing differences had been observed, but the results might have occurred by chance. In the Finnish trial, however, clear-cut effects that readily passed statistical muster could be observed for both coronary heart disease events and total mortality.

Unfortunately, the trial reached exactly the opposite of the outcome that was expected. The excess deaths and additional heart attacks were not found in the untreated control group. Instead, they occurred among those whose cholesterol and blood pressure levels had been reduced. Over the entire 15-year period the difference in mortality was alarming: a 46 percent excess, with 67 deaths occurring among those treated compared with 46 in the control group. The straightforward interpretation was that treating the high blood pressure and elevated cholesterol of 610 men had killed 21 of them. Several factors might limit the extent to which these lethal effects might be generalized to predict excess deaths among millions now being similarly treated. This trial measured the combined effects of treatment of two risk factors, not the treatment of cholesterol alone; different drugs might produce different outcomes; and finally, the subjects were observed for 15 years but treated aggressively for only 5.

Were this the only example of excess deaths in cholesterol-lowering treatment, the Finnish Multifactor Trial might be dismissed as a fluke, even though it meets all commonly accepted scientific standards. However, excess deaths have been reported with disturbing frequency in trials involving cholesterol lowering. The World Health Organization's clinical trial involving the widely prescribed drug clofibrate had produced evidence of a 29 percent excess of deaths in the treatment group. The National Heart, Lung, and Blood Institute had hastily canceled its trial of a cholesterol-lowering thyroid hormone, citing the fear that it would demonstrate the same result. It was certainly conceivable that the national programs actively promoting cholesterol-lowering treatment might be causing excess deaths instead of saving lives.

According to medical journal custom around the world, important research such as the Finnish study often warrant a separate editorial, interpreting and sometimes enlarging on the findings. Such editorials usually express an authoritative view, but necessarily the official opinion of management, as do newspaper editorials. Nevertheless it was a particularly delicate assignment, since the American Medical Association had launched its own high-profile "War on Cholesterol," urging its physician members to be more aggressive in treatment. A quarter of a million dollars to finance the AMA campaign had come from Merck, the drug company that was marketing a major cholesterol-lowering drug, lovastatin (or Mevacor). Merck also advertised lavishly in the association's journal. And the AMA had taken another $500,000 from two food companies who stood to benefit from the campaign. The job of explaining the excess deaths in the Finnish trial fell to one of the most influential proponents of risk factor epidemiology, Charles H. Hennekens of Harvard University, and a medical colleague, Oglesby Paul.

The 1,500-word article represented an extraordinary exercise in avoiding the central facts of the matter.★ The editorial meanders on for 496 words before even mentioning the trial for the first time. Meanwhile the authors discuss smoking, exercise, thrombolytic therapy, diabetes, arterial spasms, myocardial perfusion and other factors that make coronary heart disease so baffling. Finally they confess, "Perhaps we have had too high expectations." The authors do ultimately reach for a larger perspective and mention a recent analysis of six other important cholesterol-lowering trials, published in the *British Medical Journal*. But they neglect to mention the principal finding of that analysis: taken together the other six clinical trials showed cholesterol lowering had no effect on total mortality or life expectancy. The larger picture from 25 years of clinical trials was that the benefits of cholesterol lowering were so small that the slightest unexpected adverse effects of treatment could outweigh any positive risk reduction—as apparently happened in the Finnish trial. However, Hennekens and Paul preferred to insist that the contrary is true, concluding, "The totality of evidence indicated that intervention on coronary risk factors will in fact decrease the risk of cardiovascular disease." They cited as supporting evidence the National Institutes of Health's crusade against high cholesterol, modeled on its earlier war on high blood pressure. Coordinated by an NIH division called the National Heart, Lung, and Blood Institutes, it is called the National Cholesterol Education Program, and it urges medical treatment of 38 percent of the adult population. Henneken's citation of the blueprint for the nation's massive medical treatment program seemed to suggest that, of course, the health authorities could not possibly have launched such an initiative without overwhelming evidence. A review of the scientific record demonstrates that is decidedly not the case.

★The trial and full editorial are recommended reading. As with other sources for this book, a specific citation appears in the chapter notes.

. . .

The distant observer would find it strange indeed that so many people would come to fear cholesterol, an organic chemical central to the functioning of all animal cells. It is a substance so indispensable to life that every cell in the human body can manufacture it. As every high-school biology student learns, the human body is 56 percent water and combined with many chemicals that are readily soluble in water—such as sodium, calcium, potassium and sugar. But humans would be little more than an inert kettle of primordial soup were not these fluids mostly confined within 75 trillion discrete and separately functioning cells. The living boundaries of these cells—the gates of life itself—are the cell membranes. They are constructed out of cholesterol and fat compounds called lipids.

The body's specialized chemical factory, the liver, can manufacture enormous quantities of cholesterol and supplement its output with additional quantities absorbed from the blood through special receptors. Much of the liver's output of cholesterol is incorporated into bile acid, which is used to facilitate the digestion of foods containing fats. The functions of the separate cells are coordinated through the chemical messengers or hormones—many of which are built from cholesterol compounds. Sex hormones, for example. The greatest concentration of cholesterol, however, is found in the brain, where the electrical pulses ripple along filamentous nerve cell membranes, forming the signals that we perceive as thoughts, sights, sounds and smells.

At any given time, a large quantity of cholesterol circulates through the blood. Every pint of blood contains about one-third of an ounce, by weight, of cholesterol. In more conventional metric measure, every tenth of a liter (deciliter) of blood contains roughly 210 milligrams of cholesterol, although adult levels typically range from about 140 mg/dl to 340 mg/dl, and even more extreme values are occasionally observed. Unlike body temperature, cholesterol levels are not inherently stable and fluctuate by large amounts over the short term—sometimes by as much as 50 mg/dl. In the world of cholesterol hype and mass medical treatment, many unwary physicians or their patients have mistaken these random fluctuations for the results of diet or drug interventions.

However, like many vital substances, cholesterol can accumulate in undesired ways or places. It can precipitate to form crystals in the gallbladder, where supplies of the cholesterol-rich bile acid are stored. Larger crystals—or gallstones, in the common term—can be acutely painful and require surgery.

Cholesterol compounds can also be found accumulating in the damaged areas of the arteries where, in some individuals, irregular growths or lesions begin to form with advancing age. The inner walls of arteries are designed to be superslick surfaces to facilitate the passage of blood cells and the hundreds of proteins circulating in the blood. Given the ubiquitous presence of cholesterol, it is not surprising to find it accumulates in areas of the arterial walls where these lesions form. Should such lesions obstruct the network of tiny arteries that nourish the heart muscle with blood, it is a specialized case of the larger degenerative process called atherosclerosis, and given the separate medical name of coronary heart disease. Such lesions are commonplace in adults. While the numbers have never been reliably estimated, lesions could occur among 30 to 75 percent of all adults.

The lesions of coronary heart disease may be harmless and go undetected throughout life. It is possible to obstruct 75 percent of the diameter of one of the small coronary arteries without even reducing the total flow. If the heart muscle cells can get blood from nearby blood vessels, an artery can be entirely obstructed without harm, provided this occurs slowly. At autopsies conducted after accidental deaths, completely occluded arteries are frequently observed in otherwise vigorous individuals.

No one, however, would suggest this process is beneficial to health. By analogy, this degenerative mechanism is something like owning a car whose braking power is slowly and gradually eroding over a long period. Damage might be observed with inspection on the brake linings of rather new cars. Over time many drivers might not detect a slight loss of braking power, but instead instinctively hit the brakes a little earlier. Others might consciously drive more carefully and deliberately, intentionally compensating for the increasingly limited stopping ability. A majority of cars, in this analogy, hit the scrap heap for other failures before the declining brake capacity becomes an important problem. However, sometimes the brakes fail suddenly—causing death instantly.

Or in certain emergency circumstances, the diminished stopping ability robs the driver of a safety margin needed to avoid disaster.

In heart disease, also, the prime focus has logically been to prevent the accidents. The most familiar of these mishaps is the heart attack. The exact sequence of events is not certain, but a blood clot suddenly forms in a coronary artery at a location already narrowed by a lesion, and this abruptly interdicts the flow of blood to an area of heart muscle tissue. Deprived of oxygen and nutrients, the irreplaceable heart cells die. However, from one-third to one-half of coronary heart disease deaths are linked to an entirely different mechanism in which the role of the lesions remains uncertain. The heart muscle contractions are triggered by rhythmic electrical pulses that ripple in waves across the surfaces of the cell membranes. Somehow these orderly waves become disrupted, and the muscle cells twitch chaotically. No blood is therefore pumped. Sudden death is the result. In one out of five sudden-death cases, no trace of the lesions that underlie heart attacks can be found. However, in a majority of cases, lesions are present. But their role in triggering sudden death is unknown. Thus, the two most dangerous events are only indirectly related to the underlying process: one is a blood clot accident, the other an electrical disturbance.

This brief survey of the biology of coronary heart disease is intended to illustrate a key point about cholesterol lowering. Given an extremely complicated degenerative process that may be harmless in many cases, it should not be surprising that altering cholesterol levels by a small amount might have little effect on the two major disease events, sudden death and heart attack. Cholesterol is not some bacterial invader or a toxic chemical to be neutralized or destroyed, it is a substance central to numerous life processes. It is equally self-evident that altering cholesterol levels and therefore lipid metabolism could easily have negative as well as positive effects. Therefore, the results of the Finnish trial should not come as a complete surprise; the real surprise was that cholesterol should have become the centerpiece of heart disease prevention in the first place. A key step in that process occurred in a crowded auditorium at the National Institutes of Health in Bethesda, Maryland, in December 1985.

With most of the work completed for a doctoral degree in nutrition science, Beverly Teeters had a special interest in the scientific forum that was going to consider the role of diet and cholesterol in coronary heart disease. It had been proposed that animal fat and cholesterol in the diet cause coronary heart disease, and Teeters was an expert in the biochemical processes involving those and other substances. Although the American Heart Association had proclaimed for many years that diet played a key role in heart disease, Teeters, studying at the University of Maryland, was not so sure. She was therefore most interested in a forum where some of the best-known experts in the world would debate the question. Ultimately a panel would judge the evidence presented and issue conclusions that would be regarded throughout medicine and science as authoritative. The Consensus Conference on Lowering Cholesterol to Prevent Heart Disease was about to begin.

But first, a genuine accident of fate was about to occur. Teeters had missed connections with an associate from another university. She stopped at the registration desk to find the name of the hotel where the colleague was staying. Almost without thinking, she wrote the information on some paper she picked up from the registration desk. Later, she would discover she had by accident used the blank side of a document she had surely never been intended to receive. Because here, stamped "draft," were the conclusions that were going to be reached by the consensus panel before any of the evidence had even been presented. If anyone had any doubt that this conference was intended to reach only those conclusions orchestrated by the organizer—the National Heart, Lung, and Blood Institute—this was awfully persuasive evidence. It is only in the most intellectually bankrupt of issue forums that the findings are written prior to the evidence being presented. Later in the conference, major world authorities on heart disease asked to file a minority report and accused the organizers of misstating the scientific record. They were informed that such dissent was not allowed at consensus conferences. Other critics complained that the conference's clarion call for the mass treatment of elevated cholesterol would be prohibitively expensive. They were informed that such proceedings never addressed questions of cost. When key scientific judgments and pivotal health-policy decisions are made in this manner can it be any wonder that the risk factor approach to longevity has proved to be such a disappointment?

The orchestrated conclusions of the consensus conference marked a sea change at the National Heart, Lung, and Blood Institute. The drug industry had been independently promoting cholesterol-lowering treatment since 1960; given the industry's power, money and access to physicians, they had enjoyed substantial success. The American Heart Association had pushed for a big treatment program. But now, the United States government's medical research organization was going to add its weight, prestige, political and media clout to launch a bandwagon that would roll forward with astonishing speed. There were billions of dollars in the balance. Cholesterol treatment would become one of the most important new markets for prescription drugs in decades. Billions of dollars in food company sales were at stake, with major winners and losers.

The National Heart, Lung, and Blood Institute set the treatment thresholds so low that it created health anxieties in a majority of the population. With average cholesterol levels in the nation at roughly 215 mg/dl, the institute declared that any level over 200 was "borderline high" and might require treatment if other risk factors were present. Even though the elderly had average cholesterol levels of approximately 230 mg/dl, levels above 240 mg/dl were declared so dangerous that an immediate medical treatment program was advised. The net result was that 38 percent of the adult population would be dispatched to their doctors for a lifetime program of cholesterol treatment. With medical dissent effectively suppressed at the consensus conference, the promotion of cholesterol treatment rolled forward without restraint.

This heavy-handed approach, however, does not automatically mean the National Heart, Lung, and Blood Institute was wrong about the importance of cholesterol. Nor should one conclude that cholesterol lowering is pointless under all circumstances. The deeply flawed process through which this program was launched does, however, provide an important reason to look beyond authoritative medical declarations and examine the scientific evidence and the theories that evidence was intended to test. Advocacy of the treatment of high cholesterol levels— the most prominent of the risk factors—was a conscious and deliberate result of using epidemiology to attack a complex degenerative process.

In the beginning, it seemed like a perfectly logical idea. A group of farsighted medical researchers had devised a bold but carefully thought out strategy to combat a rising tide of coronary heart disease deaths observed after the close of World War II. First they would identify the risk factors associated with that disease in an epidemiological study—following in the footsteps of John Snow's discoveries about cholera and Joseph Goldberger's examination of pellagra. Next they would make certain the same risk factors could be identified in other epidemiological studies. The simplest test of the validity of such risk factor relationships is that they be found consistently in repeated studies. Finally, and most important, the validity of the risk factors would be confirmed by clinical trials measuring the effects of intervention. The investigators—at least some of them—did not intend to simply assume that if elevated blood cholesterol was associated with increased risk of coronary heart disease, lowering cholesterol would inevitably produce health benefits. The plan was to find out and measure with objective, clinical trials what actually happened when cholesterol—or blood pressure—levels were reduced. This was a bold and logical program of scientific research and, if conducted properly, would take literally decades to complete.

In the first step—an epidemiological investigation of coronary heart disease—researchers recruited two-thirds of the adult population of Framingham, Massachusetts, to become their living laboratory. From that famous study emerged four important risk factors for coronary heart disease. Age was by far the most important influence—vulnerability rose dramatically with advancing years, especially after about age 50. Then came sex. Before menopause, the Framingham data showed, women were practically immune. The researchers, however, were interested in modifiable risk factors, and so the next two influences they identified were not so important as age and sex, but they looked like they could be modified. Those factors were high blood pressure and elevated cholesterol, of which high blood pressure looked more important. Cigarette smoking was also associated with greater risk—but its influence on coronary heart disease was nowhere as compelling as its links to lung cancer—where risks were 10 to 20 times higher among heavy smokers. Smoking seemed to increase the risk for coronary heart disease by approximately 1.4 times.

Especially when considering cholesterol, it is essential to remember that a "risk factor" describes a statistical association that can be, as a practical matter, quite weak. Age, for example, is a compelling risk factor of impressive power. It so dominates the heart disease picture that 85 percent of the deaths occur in the population over age 65. More than half occur in the 15 percent of the adult population that is over age 74. And a large fraction occurs over age 80. Cholesterol, on the other hand, meets the definition of a risk factor—but the relationship is much weaker. It was not a risk factor among the women in the Framingham study before age 55. The association weakens greatly with advancing age. A majority of heart disease deaths will occur among those with about average cholesterol levels—because large elevations of cholesterol are relatively rare and heart disease is not. After age 48, the Framingham study showed, there was no relationship between cholesterol level and life expectancy. Thus, the cholesterol link was strongest in the minority of young and middle-aged men with notably elevated cholesterol levels—roughly 280 mg/dl or higher. In this small group the risk of coronary heart disease was three or four times higher than in a similar population with below-average levels. Fortunately, there were not many such people. (For example, in one later experiment it was necessary to screen 480,000 middle-aged men to find just 3,806 suitable participants for a clinical trial of individuals with cholesterol over 265 mg/dl.)

The next step in the long-term assault on heart disease was to make sure that the risk factors identified in Framingham were confirmed in other epidemiological studies. Cholesterol passed this second hurdle, when the findings were readily observed in other epidemiological studies. Cholesterol was a risk factor, the association consistently found, but it was hardly a powerful one.

All this was quite clear to researchers by the early 1960s, but the most important question remained unanswered. Would intervention work? Would lowering cholesterol levels prevent heart disease? As was seen earlier, when that issue was finally addressed with blood pressure, lowering blood pressure proved to have little or no effect on coronary heart disease, and could be harmful under some circumstances. Early on, the National Heart, Lung, and Blood Institute provided a healthy restraining influence—and agreed to sponsor and pay for large and expensive intervention trials to determine the effects of cholesterol lowering.

Not everyone in the medical community was so careful. A cholesterol-lowering drug called triparanol was declared the most important clinical advance of the year 1961, and marketed aggressively to physicians. A cholesterol-lowering thyroid hormone, dextrothyroxine, was often prescribed for recent heart attack victims. These drugs did lower cholesterol levels effectively, and their manufacturers—and many influential medical researchers—were content to assume that they must therefore prevent heart attacks. In this case, they were embarrassingly wrong. Triparanol was hastily withdrawn from the market when it turned out to have unacceptably toxic side effects. When the effects of the thyroid hormone were actually tested in an intervention trial, it had the opposite effect expected: if anything it appeared to increase the likelihood of heart attacks rather than reduce it. The biggest fiasco occurred with clofibrate, which caused 29 percent more deaths among those treated. In the year this was discovered, 1978, more than 3.6 million prescriptions were written for clofibrate in the United States, suggesting that thousands of deaths might have occurred from taking this drug. These embarrassing events received little public or media attention, but they spoke eloquently to the need to judge cholesterol lowering on the basis of intervention trials, and not rely on risk factors identified in the Framingham and other epidemiological studies, or the proclamations of drug companies and overeager health activists.

Using diet rather than drugs to lower cholesterol was a strategy that appealed to many heart disease researchers. It seemed safer and easier. By the late 1950s, Edward Ahrens had already conducted experiments in his lab at Rockefeller University that showed substituting vegetable oil for the animal fat in the controlled diet of a small group of volunteers in fact lowered their cholesterol levels. On the other hand, if you studied the diet of the Framingham subjects, those with coronary heart disease had the same diet as those who did not. The only difference that could be observed was that those without coronary heart disease tended to consume more alcohol. This makes it even more important to be guided by the results of actual intervention trials, since most epidemiological studies simply do not support the diet hypothesis. Fortunately, many such experiments have been conducted over 25 years' time. Here are the largest and most important that focused on diet or had a diet component:

Intervention Trial	Result	Year
Veterans Administration	failed	1969
Minnesota Coronary Survey	failed	1989
MRFIT	failed	1982
U.S. Heart–Diet	canceled	1971
WHO Multifactor	failed	1983
Gothenburg	failed	1986
Oslo	succeeded	1981

(See chapter notes for journal citations.)

As the table makes clear, the scientific record is one of repeated failure to reduce the number of heart attacks experienced by those treated with a cholesterol-lowering diet. However, the reasons for failure varied widely. The Minnesota Coronary Survey, for example, achieved substantial cholesterol lowering among mental hospital inmates, but had no effect on coronary heart disease, possibly because the typical patient dieted for just over one year. The Veterans Administration trial came close to succeeding, and is sometimes misquoted as having done so. (Investigators claimed to have achieved a measurable result by including strokes in the event totals after the fact. This illustrates a second unfortunate trend that occurs repeatedly in cholesterol experiments: if you don't succeed, change the definition of success.) The World Health Organization and Gothenburg trials never achieved enough cholesterol lowering to truly test the diet intervention theory. This demonstrates how difficult it is to use a diet as a medical treatment, but does not reflect on whether such a diet might work among those willing to comply faithfully over a lifetime. In terms of design, the U.S. Heart-Diet trial looked promising following a lengthy pilot study. But the National Heart, Lung, and Blood Institute was not optimistic about its prospects for success and refused to fund it.

In an effort to rewrite this history of repeated failure, cholesterol crusaders sometimes cite two other efforts that claimed success. Coronary heart disease rates fell in North Karelia, Finland, following an intensive community program to reduce smoking and change the diet. But heart disease deaths also fell simultaneously in parts of Finland where no such campaign was conducted. A trial in Finnish mental hospitals, somewhat similar to the Minnesota experiment, is sometimes cited. But this deeply flawed experiment did not even have a control group.

The bona fide success story, however, is the Oslo trial. Unlike the Finnish mental hospital experiment, it meets normally accepted scientific standards. The difference between the two treatment groups, however, was primarily explained by 9 sudden or unexplained deaths—the kind of coronary events where the link with the underlying disease process is not clear. Also, the initial cholesterol levels were exceptionally high, 328 mg/dl. This is higher than 99 percent of the United States population. The total number of coronary events apparently prevented—just 17—is so small that a diagnostic error in just 2 events would change the overall outcome from success to failure. Nevertheless, by commonly accepted principles, it worked. However, common sense says these fragile findings have little practical significance without confirming results from larger trials in a more typical population. Such evidence does not exist.

The overall results of the intervention trials prove that prospects are extremely poor for achieving a measurable reduction in coronary heart disease events through diet. It was thus extraordinary that the National Heart, Lung, and Blood Institute urged the nation's physicians to prescribe such a diet as a medical treatment for elevated cholesterol, telling doctors: "Diet is the cornerstone of treatment of high-risk cholesterol levels. The view that diet modification is impractical or doomed to failure for most patients is not justified." In moderation, lowering the fat and increasing the fiber in the American diet is a perfectly sensible idea. But given this scientific record on medical intervention, making diet a treatment prescribed by physicians, with the results monitored with cholesterol tests, is a policy certain to fail.

More conclusive answers on the effects of cholesterol lowering may be observed in intervention studies using drugs. Unfortunately, both worse and better outcomes have been reported. As noted earlier, three drug trials reported that excess deaths occurred among those treated. Despite being an assault on a killer disease, no trial to prevent coronary events in individuals who are free of disease has ever reduced deaths in the period during which the drugs were being administered. This is not a treatment that saves lives.

On the benefits side, however, reduced numbers of nonfatal heart attacks have been repeatedly observed in drug trials, even in efforts that were an overall failure. The WHO trial of clofibrate—which caused excess deaths—reported fewer nonfatal heart attacks. The United States Coronary Drug Project reported fewer subsequent nonfatal heart attacks among heart attack survivors who took large doses of the vitamin niacin. The trial investigators reported the outcome as a failure because of lack of expected impact on mortality. A National Heart, Lung, and Blood Institute trial involving the drug cholestyramine (or Questran) came close to demonstrating a small reduction in heart attacks (another case where a claim of beneficial results was achieved only by changing the definition of success after the fact).

The most successful of all prevention trials—one using the drug gemfibrozil (or Lopid)—reduced the number of coronary events overall. To judge the benefits of cholesterol lowering over five years' time, it is therefore helpful to examine the results of this success story directly.

HELSINKI TRIAL

	Treatment	Placebo
Subjects	2,051	2,030
Heart attacks	51	79
Sudden death	5	4
Total deaths (all causes)	45	42

These results can be portrayed in dramatically different terms. Cholesterol crusaders said a 10 percent reduction in cholesterol had achieved a 34 percent reduction in the risk of a heart attack. And on the basis of this trial, gemfibrozil has been heavily advertised in the United States, and was prescribed for at least 3.7 million people. Skeptics noted that treating more than 2,000 persons with $300,000 worth of drugs over five years' time might have prevented 28 heart attacks and saved no lives. As Alan Brett wrote in the *New England Journal of Medicine,* "How does one weigh a benefit for 14 people against the effects of treating 986 people who are not destined to benefit?" One answer is to look at the ill effects of treatment that were reported among the 986 who were not helped.

One wonders how many physicians read the fine print about side effects on the gemfibrozil circular from the manufacturer, Warner-

Lambert. It revealed that the negative trend on total mortality (originally 45 deaths in the treatment group compared with 42 in placebo) had continued with increasing follow-up (59 deaths to 55 deaths). Gemfibrozil is a close chemical cousin of the ill-fated clofibrate. The circular says, "This result is not statistically significantly different from the 29 percent excess mortality seen in the clofibrate group in the WHO study." Another similarity to clofibrate was an increased incidence of gallstones, "a 55 percent excess." In fact, treatment was more likely to cause gallstones than to prevent nonfatal heart attacks.

There was another problem. These meager benefits, and frequent side effects, were being observed in a specific high-risk population—middle-aged men with large elevations of cholesterol. This was the population where epidemiological studies had shown the strongest link with coronary heart disease. It ought, therefore, to be of great concern to discover that gemfibrozil and other cholesterol-lowering drugs were being prescribed mainly for other populations, where the cholesterol link to heart disease was weak, suspect, nonexistent or undetermined. For example, 55 percent of the cholesterol-lowering drug prescriptions in 1988 were for women, for whom no clinical trial evidence of benefit existed; among younger women the cholesterol relationship was not even found in epidemiological studies. Fifty-nine percent of the prescriptions were being written for those over age 60. The cholesterol relationship weakens dramatically with age, and the benefits of cholesterol lowering had never been tested in this group. Given that it was not absolutely clear that benefits outweigh harm even in the narrowly selected population of young and middle-aged men with severe elevations of cholesterol, the medical authorities were taking a grave risk promoting treatment in large subgroups where benefits were unknown and treatment might be harmful to health.

The 25 years during which cholesterol-lowering treatments had been tested had brought a steady lowering of expectations for what they should accomplish. In the mid-1960s, a major trial was designed with a cholesterol-lowering diet of a typical duration of two years or less. When it resulted in no effects, researchers concluded it must take more time to demonstrate benefits. In the 1970s, investigators expected to reduce deaths in recent heart attack victims treated for five years. When this failed, they concluded that maybe total mortality wasn't the right measure of benefits after all, and began to focus on nonfatal heart attacks. The trials reported in the 1980s lasted up to 7.5 years and produced a few successes (such as the Helsinki trial), but the researchers didn't even hope to produce evidence of saving lives with treatment. Trials were lasting longer and longer; they required thousands of volunteers and took more than a decade from design to final report—and even then most experiments failed or produced marginal results.

All this was in stark contrast to the dazzling power of effective medical treatments. With penicillin for raging pneumonia infection, or diuretics to combat malignant high blood pressure, it was quite possible to demonstrate effectiveness immediately with just two patients. The treated patient would survive and the untreated subject would die. It didn't take observing thousands of people over many years in hopes of demonstrating 20 or 30 had benefited. To those who probed beneath the hype of health-promotion propaganda, the arithmetic of medical treatment to lower cholesterol was dismal.

In the late 1980s, as doubts were quietly mounting, a new benefit of cholesterol lowering was aggressively publicized: regression of coronary heart disease. With drastic cholesterol lowering of 20 percent or more, investigators reported that some of the lesions that underlie the degenerative process of coronary heart disease had shrunk or disappeared. What more powerful proof could anyone ask that cholesterol lowering worked! While it took a one-two punch of powerful drugs, some of the irregular growths in the arteries appeared to be actually melting away. Here was a treatment that claimed to "reverse" coronary heart disease. The National Heart, Lung, and Blood Institute heavily promoted this new success, a trial with 184 subjects called the Cholesterol Lowering Atherosclerosis Study, or CLAS. As usual, few hard questions were asked or answered.

The CLAS study differed strikingly from all previous clinical trials. A major limitation of all such previous experiments was the extremely modest cholesterol lowering actually achieved—a reduction of 2 to 10 percent. In the CLAS study, cholesterol levels were reduced 26 percent. All 184 patients had advanced coronary heart disease—so there was no chance of diluting the beneficial effects by treating people who didn't have and never would get this disease. If ever treatment was going to work, achieving drastic cholesterol change in subjects with extremely serious cases ought to do the trick. Finally, the investigators were going to examine the condition of the coronary arteries directly, by flooding them with a radioactive dye and monitoring the results with x-ray pictures. The pictures were the source of the most heavily promoted finding.

After just two years' treatment, the investigators reported "16.2 percent of the drug subjects vs. 2.3 percent of the placebo subjects showed regression." By "regression" they meant the lesions obstructing the arteries were getting smaller, instead of becoming slowly and irreversibly larger. While this failed to occur in 84 percent of the patients thus treated, benefiting even 14 percent (2.3 percent improved without treatment) might constitute a dramatic improvement over previous trials, where at best only 1–2 percent were benefited. Finally, this was only a two-year trial. Should this rollback continue over time, think of the possible benefits after five years! This is how it looked to the optimists and health promoters who badly needed evidence that the vast cholesterol treatment program they had launched was producing real benefits.

In fact, the CLAS study "succeeded" only by employing a new definition of success—reporting what was occurring inside the coronary arteries, not whether the subjects were living healthier or longer lives. "Regression," which sounds so dramatic, was in fact defined as any "perceptible change" in the shape of the growths. However, if one looked at the outcome that would concern most patients—a major adverse medical event—the results were quite different.

CLAS
MAJOR ADVERSE MEDICAL EVENTS

	Treatment	Placebo
Subjects	92	92
Cardiovascular events	25	24
Sudden death	0	1
Other events	18	7
Total	43	32

The combination of large doses of two very powerful cholesterol-lowering drugs (colestipol and niacin) was unmistakably causing major adverse health events—grouped together in the table above as "Other events." These included gastrointestinal disorders, gout, liver and urological abnormalities—all established side effects of the drugs. On the plus side, therefore, among 92 participants in the trial, apparently 12 patients had lesions that "perceptibly improved"—a change that would be completely undetectable to the patient. However, 18 suffered major adverse medical events, and another 25 suffered the kind of cardiovascular event treatment was intended to prevent. These are only the major events. If less-severe side effects of treatment are included, there were 91 percent who experienced flushing or other skin irregularities (typical side effects of niacin) and large numbers of gastrointestinal problems (typical complications of colestipol): constipation (31 percent), heartburn (20 percent), abdominal pain (15 percent), sore throat (14 percent) and vomiting (6 percent). It was a sad testimony about what really happens to patients receiving intensive cholesterol-lowering treatment. Of the 92 patients treated, 47 percent had suffered a major adverse medical event in just two years' time, and practically all had side effects, and some, multiple side effects. Such was the breakthrough success in which "regression" of coronary heart disease was first detected.

It was not until November 1990 that an answer was provided for the last critical question about cholesterol lowering. Would the modest amount of "regression" observed after two years in the CLAS trial increase dramatically over greater intervals of time? Were the 14 percent of the lesions that shrank just the beginning of a slowly moving rollback of this disease that might be achieved over five or ten years? The answer could be found in the longest and most unusual clinical trial in the annals of heart disease research. In this case cholesterol lowering was achieved through a major surgical procedure that created a shortcut through the long, twisting coils of the intestine. Through bypassing a portion of the intestine, the absorption of all foods consumed was drastically reduced, especially dietary cholesterol. As a result, cholesterol levels fell dramatically, by 23 percent on the average. All the subjects participating had advanced heart disease, and they were observed for 9.7 years. Since this was a surgical procedure, compliance—the other problem with all risk factor disease treatments—was perfect. Furthermore, the investigators directly examined the condition of the coronary arteries every two years as in the CLAS trial. This experiment—the Partial Ileal Bypass Trial—provides the authoritative answer to whether regression was an important effect.

This much larger (838 patients) and longer trial failed to detect any significant effects on regression. "The rate of regression in the treatment group exceeded that in the control group," the investigators reported. "However, this apparent regression may represent random variation." After 10 continuous years of cholesterol-lowering effects, regression was detected in 6 percent of the treated patients and 3.8 percent of the untreated control group. The trial also failed to reach its intended objective, reducing total mortality.

Over 10 years' time, the investigators claimed to have prevented 43 events—nonfatal and fatal heart attacks. To achieve this outcome they had conducted major surgery on 421 persons. Another 15 required a second major operation to remove bowel obstructions caused by the initial surgery, and 42 others required medical treatment for a bowel obstruction. An additional 14 patients required major surgery to remove gallstones— another complication of cholesterol lowering. And 40 others had less-severe gallstones that didn't yet need surgery. Every year 4 percent of the surgery group got painful kidney stones. The investigators don't provide a grand total, but a simple calculation suggests that perhaps 200 patients suffered this unpleasant problem over the 10 years. Another 6 to 8 percent had constantly recurring diarrhea. Virtually none of the control group experienced these complications. When reported in November 1991, the study's chief investigator, University of Minnesota surgeon Henry Buchwald, launched a national publicity blitz proclaiming this trial was the most convincing proof yet of the benefits of cholesterol lowering.

How could reputable medical scientists promote cholesterol-lowering medical treatment under these circumstances? They were part of a deeply flawed system that encourages and rewards such misjudgments. A powerful group of the medical elite had wagered their careers on a particular, narrow approach to preventing coronary heart disease. They also committed a large share of the National Heart, Lung, and Blood Institute's research budget to testing their theories. The same group controlled the American Heart Association, which had publicly campaigned against cholesterol for literally decades. Under these circumstances, it is not surprising that a group of researchers overcommitted to a particular approach could not read the handwriting on the wall that said, "You failed."

Thus it happened that the real pressures were to not face reality. Outside critics could be disregarded. The real pressures were to help the drug industry, where some of the large companies had also bet heavily on cholesterol. So low are the ethical standards at the National Institutes of Health that it is almost impossible to find any boundary between the government, the drug industry and the medical elite.

For example, nothing prevents lavish fees from being paid to the medical school physicians who served on the institute's advisory panels, made decisions recommending specific drug treatments, evaluated grants or monitored the safety of patients taking drugs in clinical trials.

The flavor of the lavish scale on which drug companies make payments to the medical school faculty elite could be gleaned from a new report in the *Journal of the American Medical Association*. At a meeting to discuss the problem, the drug companies apparently expressed the need for protection from the professors' cash demands. "Excesses abound on both sides," the report said, "as 'marquee professors' demand high fees and extraordinary expense accounts from pharmaceutical companies for speaking engagements at conferences."

To clean up some of the worst conflicts, one might look for leadership to the director of the National Institutes of Health, Bernadine Healy. After earlier work as a research physician on an NIH trial of an important new drug to combat heart attacks, Healy had purchased stock in the company that held the patent, Genentech, before the study was published. At the time Healy was also president of the American Heart Association, which published an important medical journal focusing on heart disease, *Circulation*. The editor of that journal at the time, Burton Sobel, was consultant to the same drug company, and received company stock options, according to a report in *The Wall Street Journal*. It was not, therefore, surprising when soon after Healy became director of NIH, she sought to curb the limited ethical enforcement activities of her mammoth health research agency.

When asked about the propriety of Healy's stock purchase, former American Heart Association president Antonio Gotto told *The Wall Street Journal* he had "no questions about her ethics." Here was an unusual case of the pot calling the kettle clean. Gotto, a senior spokesman for the American Heart Association and major architect of the war on cholesterol, had himself helped Merck promote its cholesterol-lowering drug, lovastatin. No wonder he had no difficulties with Healy's behavior.

One might occasionally see public service advertisements reminding the public of the importance of taking cholesterol-lowering drugs. They were produced by the same small "citizens" group that made so many high blood pressure advertisements, except it took a new name, Citizens for Public Action on Cholesterol. The president was Gotto. As usual, funds were collected from the drug companies.

Others seeking information about cholesterol might look to the newsletter *It's YOUR Cholesterol!* published by the lipid research unit at George Washington University Medical School. They might read an article by the clinic director, John R. LaRosa, who was also the national education chairman for the National Cholesterol Education Program. Rather than discussing excess mortality in repeated clinical trials, LaRosa would write, "Cholesterol-lowering drugs are among the safest drugs in current use and need not be feared."

The newsletter was published using money from Bristol Laboratories, which sells the cholesterol-lowering drug cholestyramine (or Questran). It was specifically recommended as the drug of choice under the National Cholesterol Education Program treatment guidelines, which LaRosa helped write. A handsome brochure urging aggressive treatment of elevated cholesterol and recommending this drug was provided to every primary-care physician in the United States.

These multiple roles and hidden priorities help explain why the public receives such an unbalanced view of the actual risks and benefits of cholesterol lowering. This is no conspiracy—but the result of a closed circle of medical insiders operating without the normal checks and ethical barriers that force closer adherence to truth in other scientific disciplines. One hopes to find drug companies, citizens groups, prominent medical researchers, and the NIH acting as checks on each other. In reality one finds a tight-knit band all playing the same song. Because the problem occurs among the institutions that conduct the medical research on cholesterol, it means that thousands of conscientious physicians receive equally biased information, and are also frequently misled. If they attend a medical conference to learn more about lipids, they will hear from an expert on the drug company payroll. Many physicians did probe beyond the cholesterol hype and read the research results. That just made their lives more difficult as they faced criticism from less-inquiring colleagues and a public that demanded to know their cholesterol levels and wanted to lower them.

In the end, the cholesterol crusade played so well because it told the public what it wanted to hear. It provided a magic longevity number, the ready assistance of reassuring experts to help make it move in the right direction. Here was another health commandment for a daily regimen of virtue. One only wishes that the researchers who launched the cholesterol crusade had understood the disease as thoroughly as they had mastered the skill to manipulate public fears.

Meanwhile, doubts about the wisdom of cholesterol treatment began to be expressed more openly in influential scientific journals. A 1992 analysis in the *British Medical Journal* cited the disappointing results of diet and the failure of drug treatment to reduce mortality even among the men at highest risk. It proposed a moratorium on the use of cholesterol-lowering drugs.

An equally far-reaching proposal to end the aggressive American cholesterol treatment program came in a September 1992 editorial in the flagship medical journal of the American Heart Association, *Circulation*.

"We need now to pull back our national policies directed at identifying and treating high blood cholesterol," wrote Steven B. Hulley and two colleagues at the University of California at San Francisco. He urged the medical community "to put on hold well meant desires to intervene while we await convincing evidence that the net effects of treatment will be beneficial."

One would have thought no responsible medical authority would have even considered promoting the medical treatment of millions of adults for high cholesterol without first having conclusive evidence of such a net benefit. One also would have thought that the treatment of high blood pressure would have been targeted only at those for whom benefits had been proven. But as was shown earlier, that was not the case either. And one would suppose that if being overweight were going to be made into a medical problem, a safe and effective medical solution must first exist. It truly is one of the great tragedies of public health policy that so much money and energy has been expended to achieve so little effect.

CHAPTER ELEVEN

WHAT'S IN YOUR GENES?

Among those who learn that modifying risk factors has minimal effect on life expectancy, one reaction is quite common. The person sighs and remarks, "It's all in our genes." Indeed, genes do play a critical role in our prospects. However, the atmosphere of resignation and fatalism that seems to accompany such declarations is not justified. To examine what is in our genes is to understand the extent to which all humans share a common set of coded instructions, secrets of life that have been preserved, edited and refined for hundreds of generations. To grasp the possibilities defined by our genes is also to observe a mechanism that provides such remarkable diversity that each of us amounts to a unique experiment. To explore the role of genes in longevity is to realize that the same set of genes might be beneficial in one environment but harmful in another. Although genes may define the rules for the game of life, they rarely determine the outcome.

The most intriguing paradox of genetics and longevity might be defined in this way: The past two decades have brought an explosion of scientific knowledge emphasizing the role of genes in a vast array of health disorders that shorten life. Specific locations have been pinpointed for juvenile-onset diabetes, Duchenne's muscular dystrophy, hemophilia, Huntington's disease, cystic fibrosis, one cause of heart disease and a rare variety of eye cancer. More speculative and still mainly statistical evidence suggests an important genetic component or predisposition for obesity, high blood pressure, colon cancer, lung cancer, alcoholism, schizophrenia, manic-depressive disorder and Alzheimer's disease. Nevertheless there is surprisingly little evidence to support the most common conception of an influential genetic role in longevity—that the lifespan of one's parents and grandparents provides a reliable indication of one's own prospects. This chapter will examine why genes can be so important, yet your parents' history be such an unreliable guide to your own future.

Another major aspect of genes will be addressed later in the book. The possibility that life expectancy is regulated by a genetic "clock" or limited by genes in other ways will be examined in the chapter that considers the possibility of achieving a quantum leap in life expectancy.

The link between one's own and a parent's longevity becomes immediately more precarious upon a brief examination of exactly how those genes are acquired. In modern usage, a gene is a specific segment of the one billion letters of DNA code that are strung along the twisted coils of the 46 chromosomes. All but two of the chromosomes are arranged in matched pairs, providing duplicate copies of most of the 50,000 to 100,000 genes. The exception is the sex-determining chromosomes, where men have only one complete copy of the entire X chromosome and one Y-shaped fragment, and women have two complete X chromosomes. This means that for most of the biological functions now understood, each individual has two genes containing the necessary code, one acquired from each parent, who in turn had two different copies.

To possess one copy of a particular gene—perhaps a longevity gene—does not necessarily mean that the gene will be expressed. Both copies could lie fallow, idle and unused because they were never switched on. One copy might be expressed and the other remain inactive. Or both might operate and interact. It depends entirely on the gene, its purpose, its matching duplicate and its function.

Unfortunately the function of only a few thousand genes is now understood. The simplest case is called a dominant gene with complete penetrance. Such a gene is always expressed if acquired from either parent. Such genes, however, are extremely rare. There are many more known cases involving recessive gene defects, which have little or no effect unless the individual inherits two flawed copies. Many genetic disorders—for example, cystic fibrosis and sickle cell anemia—occur, or become severe, only when duplicate copies of a defective gene are present. In fact, it is estimated that among the 50,000 to 100,000 genes, every person has three defective genes that would prove lethal to a descendant who inherited a second defective copy from the other parent. However, the chances of losing this game of genetic roulette are about 1 in 99. If there are recessive genes that provide longevity benefits, the odds of inheriting the necessary two copies might be similarly small.

In addition, the cells that become a sperm and an egg undergo a special form of cell division, called meosis, that creates new genetic possibilities not present in the duplicate chromosomes of the parent. One mechanism corrects errors in duplication and another may combine segments from both the duplicate chromosomes rather than simply passing on one entire chromosome. So the person who wonders if he will live as long as his mother has only half her chromosomes, and even these are not exact copies.

Despite these complexities, examples of long-lived families have been reported in the scientific and medical literature for at least 100 years. Although ingrained in folk wisdom, such cases provide a dramatic example of the dangers of being deceived by observational bias. Without systematic observation, nobody would remember the many families where long-lived grandparents had offspring with average or below-average lifespans. To complicate matters further, genes are not the only factors associated with longevity that are passed from generation to generation. Common trends in education, income, social status, residential location and even occupation are readily observed in families, and all have been associated with differences in life expectancy. Without systematic observation, the risk is great that the members of a long-lived family shared only an unusual common run of good luck.

Also, advantageous genes do not exist in the abstract like a savings account that is available for whatever needs might emerge. Except for clear biological malfunctions, such as diabetes, the exact same gene might prove an advantage or a hindrance depending on the environment. Consider the genes that determine skin color. In the United States, blacks have a life expectancy seven years shorter than whites. But it is not difficult to imagine an environment in which blacks typically outlive whites. As noted earlier, gender provided a longevity disadvantage to women throughout most of human history. Today, it provides an advantage of five years in Japan, seven years in the United States and ten years in the republics of the former Soviet Union. One would suppose the primary difference was not in the genetic endowment but in the environments in which these men and women live.

"Longevity" genes might exist. However, they could be extremely hard to identify unless they were present in a relatively large group of people and performed limited and readily identifiable biochemical functions that were beneficial over a wide variety of environmental conditions. For these reasons, the search for longevity genes must be conducted with great caution, for fear of studying long-lived families that don't have any such genes—the problem of selection bias—or overlooking genes whose benefits were concealed or offset by environmental factors.

One of the first systematic examinations of the long-lived was conducted in the 1920s by a Johns Hopkins University researcher named Raymond Pearl. From newspaper clippings and other public sources Pearl collected the names of 2,319 individuals who had reached the age of 90—a much rarer event in 1920 than today. Then he attempted to determine how long their parents and grandparents had lived. Pearl found an effect, but the study succumbs to the problem of observational bias. He only traced the complete family history of 365 individuals—and generally the forebears easiest to trace would be those who lived longest. However, thirty years later, Pearl's original longevity files formed the starting point for a much stronger effort. A team of Hopkins medical geneticists led by Margaret R. Hawkins traced the history of 9,205 offspring of the original group of 90-year-olds, locating 85 percent of their children. Hawkins reported, "There was a clear but weak trend for survival to increase with increasing age of death of the proband [starting individual under study] parent." As in many other studies, the mother's age proved more influential than the father's. However, the Hawkins study is still not persuasive evidence of heritable longevity genes: it included only offspring who already had survived to age 20, and included four decades during which national mortality rates steadily declined. Most important, it measured only the combined environmental and genetic advantages of being a member of a long-lived family.

The seamless fabric of heredity and family environment was partially unraveled in an intriguing adoption study conducted in Denmark, where a national register of adopted children is available to researchers.

It compared the influences of adoptive and biological parents on the subsequent mortality of 960 Danish children followed for 57 years after birth, focusing on the premature death of the parents.

Overall, the premature death of adoptive parents had no influence on their children's chances of also dying prematurely. (The children had only reached age 57 at the study's end.) On the other hand, the biological parents did pass on some of the risk of dying prematurely. Among the children with both biological parents still living, 9 percent had died of natural causes, compared with 17 percent of those with a parent who died before age 50. In relative terms, the excess risk of dying is roughly comparable to smoking.

The particular disease vulnerabilities that biological parents passed on to their children proved especially intriguing. The danger of premature death from infectious disease was the most powerful inherited factor. Among adoptees with both parents alive, only 3 percent died of infectious disease, compared with nearly 13 percent of adoptees with a parent who also died prematurely from some infection. Researchers found a valid but weaker relationship between premature death of biological parents and children from heart disease and stroke. No link was present for cancer, which was the single specific instance in which a measurable influence of adoptive parents was detected. The early death of an adoptive parent from cancer increased the risk for their children. In the adoptive families, however, the excess risk of cancer at these relatively early ages was not large enough to push the overall mortality higher.

The finding that vulnerability to infectious disease was the most powerful inherited influence recalls the earlier discussion about how tuberculosis declined spontaneously by killing off virtually the entire population without the genes to resist it. Consider this landmark study of twins from the heyday of tuberculosis:

Relationship	% with Tuberculosis
One-egg twin	87%
Two-egg twin	26%
Other sibling	26%
Spouse	7%

One hundred and fifty years ago the most important "longevity genes" might have been those that improved resistance to TB. Today they might be inconsequential.

Denmark contributed another landmark study of genes and longevity. An examination of every pair of twins born from 1870 to 1910 showed that the lifespan of identical twins varied by an average of 14.5 years, dramatizing the powerful influence of environmental and random events even when genes were identical and the family environment presumably similar. On the other hand, there was an even bigger difference for fraternal twins of the same sex—18.7 years, suggesting genes do play a broad but limited role.

The French population geneticist Albert Jacquard summed up the evidence on the heritability of longevity at an international conference in Rome in 1980. The effect, he concluded, may be present but it is small. To paraphrase his more technical conclusions, one could say that by knowing how long someone's parents lived it might be possible to predict that individual's life expectancy 2.6 percent more accurately than by simply assuming his or her lifespan would be average. "In other words, environmental factors are so important . . . that genetic factors seem insignificant by comparison," said Jacquard. This does not, however, undermine the importance of genes. It only means the diversity is too great; not only are we all different biologically, we live in different environments. And as was noted earlier, it is likely that the force of evolution selects for individuals who reproduce more effectively, with at best uncertain effects after the reproductive years. Will your lifespan resemble your parents'? Such simple propositions can be valid only in a vastly simpler world than the one in which we live.

Under certain but rare circumstances, however, the power of specific genes over longevity can be awesome. For example, some individuals carry killer genes, lurking quietly in the DNA until age 40, when they blossom to trigger neurological decline and death. It is likely there are longevity genes—and at least one specific candidate has already been identified. And between these extremes are a broad array of specific genes likely but not certain to influence life expectancy.

To identify such important effects for specific genes does not, as it might seem, conflict with the previous finding that parental genes do not accurately predict longevity overall. Some genes are present in too small a fraction of the population to influence the overall average. Millions of people carry recessive genes—either damaging or possibly beneficial—that are not activated unless some descendant acquires two copies during the genetic roulette of creation. Other genes create an opportunity for benefit or harm, but the enabling events never occur. For example, a gene that might provide more efficient oxygen absorption at high altitudes might have no effect on a family whose descendants lived near sea level on a coastal plain. Still others are tradeoff genes, helpful or harmful depending on environmental conditions. Modern-day blacks regard sickle cell anemia as a harmful genetic defect; theoretically it may have been an advantage in the malaria-infested zones of Africa where the trait originated. Genes predisposing people toward obesity may have been harmless under conditions where food supplies were scarce and advantageous if food were available only at erratic intervals.

Huntington's disease provides a clear and tragic example of a mysterious killer gene. Victims undergo progressive mental deterioration, personality change and involuntary muscle movements, ending in premature death. A single copy of the gene acquired from either parent causes the onset of the disease, with the first symptoms typically appearing after age 40. It probably originated from a mutation in a single European individual a few centuries ago.

It is a newcomer compared, for example, with the gene for a blood protein called globin, which evolution has preserved identically in many species of animal without significant change for 500 million years. A 306-letter sequence that codes for the protein histone can be found in humans, cows and pea plants, and has been preserved without change for 1 to 2 billion years. Useful genetic information about biological processes is preserved perfectly for periods so long that in the interim mountain ranges rise and are worn away, and entire continents migrate across the ocean. Other genes vary so widely among individuals that no basis exists to define which is "normal."

The newcomer, Huntington's, is quite rare—with 25,000 persons in the United States with symptoms and perhaps 125,000 individuals in families who may carry the gene. Why such a destructive mutation has survived is an object lesson in the interactions between the random choices of genetics and the blind force of evolution. First, the onset of the disease symptoms typically does not occur until after the reproductive years. Such a rare mutation still might have died out except that, prior to symptoms appearing, it increases sex drive. Therefore, Huntington's disease victims produce higher-than-average numbers of offspring and a killer gene survives.

A dominant gene with certain onset also made Huntington's an ideal early target for DNA researchers trying to perfect better techniques to find exactly where among the one billion letters of genetic code in every human cell the segment that codes for a specific gene might be located. And with Huntington's disease, they achieved an important success. This dramatic breakthrough was ably narrated by Jerry E. Bishop and Michael Waldholz in their recent book, *Genome*. What was learned—and still remains unknown—also is a lesson in the potential and limitations of current knowledge of the genetic code.

To search for such errors—which might be additions, deletions or incorrect letters—is a daunting task. Each cell contains the equivalent in genetic code of a 100-volume encyclopedia. The problem might be as minor as one letter misplaced in a short sequence. The search must be conducted without an index, table of contents, chapter headings, paragraphs or other shortcuts. The main landmarks are a handful of locations where other genes have already been pinpointed, the fruits of all previous genetic research.

One task, however, can be executed quite efficiently. Long stretches of DNA in two individuals can be compared, revealing whether they are identical. It's like owning a machine that will quickly compare two pages of text and report whether they are exactly alike, but no other information. Therefore, the search for Huntington's genes begins with slicing the DNA code of two individuals—one normal and one with the disorder—into thousands of segments, in hopes of eventually locating two pieces of DNA that are always different in individuals with the disease.

The key, therefore, is dividing the genome into segments to compare—and this is the special capability of a group of proteins called restriction enzymes. They are produced by many bacteria, and have the unique ability to sever a segment of DNA at only a particular, specific sequence of genetic code, usually from three to twenty letters long. In bacteria they function like an immune system to slice up alien DNA into nonfunctional pieces. (Meanwhile, the bacteria's own DNA is guarded by a special coat of carbon and hydrogen molecules shaped to block the enzyme.) Researchers have catalogued numerous such enzymes that will consistently sever the chromosomes at particular locations.

The breakthrough in the search for a Huntington's gene occurred almost immediately when one such enzyme, known as HindIII, was used. It was being employed to slice segments of DNA on the fourth chromosome of an individual with normal DNA and a Huntington's victim. Imagine comparing two similar volumes of an encyclopedia for errors. The text will be divided into segments at every occurrence of a particular sequence of letters. At one location on chromosome 4 the enzyme invariably located that sequence and severed the DNA in normal individuals. But in Huntington's victims it did not. It was a remarkable stroke of good fortune that the error happened to fall in a 13-letter sequence used by the enzyme HindIII. That was the unique gift of a protein manufactured by a bacterium that otherwise occupies itself multiplying in the upper respiratory tract of young children. It is like beginning a search for one typographical error in the encyclopedia and finding it at the top of the page arbitrarily picked as a beginning point.

Good fortune, however, has its limits. Nine years after the Huntington's gene was found on the fourth chromosome, researchers still do not know where the sequence begins, where it ends, or what function the gene performs. When the disease symptoms begin, the disease victims still cannot be helped.

However, those who carry the gene and will eventually develop the disease can now be identified with 95 percent certainty. Now that these genetic breakthroughs began to illuminate a whole new room of human knowledge, a new series of questions, rather than a set of wonderful answers, has emerged. The child of a parent who has developed Huntington's disease has a 50 percent chance of carrying the gene. If you are that child, do you want to know? Does a woman want to know if her fetus carries the gene? If you know you carry the gene, is your life insurance company also entitled to know before selling you a policy at the same price as others? Your employer? Your fiance? In cases—thus far quite rare—where what's in your genes unquestionably does influence life expectancy, a whole new family of problems is created.

What are the prospects when the Huntington's gene is completely characterized? The case of Duchenne's muscular dystrophy may provide some important clues. In this disorder, the muscle cells are missing a key structural protein. As a result, the muscle cells progressively weaken and die beginning in early childhood. Survival past age 20 is rare. In this instance, however, the sequence of discoveries is longer. The location of the gene was found on the X chromosome. The specific starting and ending points of the sequence were identified. Researchers learned the function of this sequence of genetic code: instructions for the manufacture of an enormous protein called dystrophin. It is missing from the muscle cells of Duchenne's muscular dystrophy patients. So far, however, this still hasn't helped the victims. The result thus far is something like the problem facing a clever engineer who stands in front of a new skyscraper he has discovered is predestined for premature collapse because a key alloy was omitted from its framework of structural steel. Having a supply of the missing alloy in his briefcase is of little immediate help.

Other genetic disorders, however, have not proved quite so intractable. Treatment was more readily devised for infants threatened with mental retardation and other ill effects from a group of disorders called PKU, or phenylketonuria. Phenylalanine is one of the eight amino acids that cannot be synthesized in the body and therefore must be obtained through diet. However, a genetic defect on chromosome 12 causes the liver to be unable to synthesize a key enzyme needed to help break down any excess quantities of the amino acid. As a result, damaging amounts of phenylalanine accumulate in the bloodstream. Since the amino acid is obtained only through diet, the condition can be managed through special foods with carefully controlled amounts of phenylalanine. Infants are routinely screened for the condition, and fetal tests can be performed.

While the number of known single-gene disorders is quite large, the fraction of the population directly affected is quite small. The latest catalogue of the human genome, *Mendelian Inheritance in Man,* lists 2,656 known locations where mutations or variations have occurred, and another 2,281 under active study. Although this totals nearly 5,000 different single-gene disorders, they are found in only 1 percent of all births, according to the 1991 edition of a major reference, the *Cecil Textbook of Medicine.*

The most widespread mutant gene causes cystic fibrosis, and is carried by 4 percent of the white population of European origin. Victims have no gene to manufacture the cell membrane channel that excretes excess chloride from lung cells. Death from respiratory causes occurs in the mid-20s. Like most of the defective genes that are well understood, cystic fibrosis is recessive, and the clinical disease does not occur except in individuals who receive defective genes from both parents. Since this occurs in only 1 out of 4 cases even when both parents have a copy of the defective gene, clinical cases of cystic fibrosis are few—roughly 30,000 in the United States.

All the defective genes thus far specifically identified are recessive genes rather than dominant. This is probably because most recessive genes are coded instructions for enzymes, the special proteins that facilitate the transformation of other proteins from one form to another—helping to either assemble more complex structures or break them down into more basic building blocks. Enzymes are easy to identify because the presence or absence of the end products can be detected. Because the body has so much natural reserve capacity, it is usually sufficient if accurate instructions for making an enzyme have survived on at least one chromosome. Dominant genes, on the other hand, cause disease in those who inherit one normal copy and one mutation. They probably perform regulatory functions rather than manufacture enzymes or structural proteins, and these processes have been much more difficult to identify and understand.

A widespread gene capable of causing early heart disease falls halfway between recessive and dominant disorders. Those with familial hypercholesterolemia, or inherited high cholesterol levels, lack either one or two copies of the gene that allows the liver to absorb cholesterol-fat compounds from the bloodstream. The liver ordinarily consumes some of the circulating cholesterol compounds as raw materials for the manufacture of other products. Since the liver, like all cells, can synthesize cholesterol on its own, its overall function is not compromised. But blood cholesterol levels in these individuals are unusually high. Individuals with one defective copy of the gene—about one half of one percent of the population—have cholesterol levels of 300 mg/dl or higher, and are at high risk for coronary heart disease in their 30s and 40s. Individuals with two defective copies have astronomical cholesterol levels—1,200 mg/dl or higher—and die of heart disease or other disorders in childhood.

Those crusading for mass treatment of high cholesterol seem to have drawn exactly the wrong conclusions from the major scientific break-through that identified the gene and its function. They have taken it as proof of the causal role of elevated cholesterol levels in coronary heart disease, but when it is examined carefully it undermines the existing evidence. Coronary pathologists have shown that the irregular growths in the arteries resulting from familial hypercholesterolemia are similar to—but by no means identical with—those in otherwise normal individuals. Just as obesity and high blood pressure are likely the measurable result of several quite different initiating disorders, coronary heart disease is a result of at least two separate and independent causes—inherited genes causing high cholesterol, and the still unknown cause in everyone else. None of the clinical trials testing cholesterol-lowering treatment and none of the epidemiological studies measuring the heart attack risks of elevations distinguished the genetic defect from the other cases. Vanderbilt University heart disease researcher George V. Mann has observed that the clinical trials are fatally flawed from failure to exclude those with the defective gene. Those with extremely high cholesterol levels are much more likely to have the gene than the rest of the population. And because the clinical trials focused on those with cholesterol levels higher than 95 percent of the population, they were likely to have attracted unusual numbers of participants with this disorder. Because of this failing, it is certain that both risk of high cholesterol and the benefits of treatment for everyone else have been overestimated. It seems quite likely that the marginal benefits of treatment analyzed earlier might disappear entirely if individuals with the genetic disorder were screened out of these studies.

It is possible that there are as many longevity genes as life-shortening mutations. However, the effects have been harder to identify, and have understandably attracted a tiny fraction of the research effort that has focused on defective genes. Thus far there has been only one candidate for a life-prolonging gene, but it is a provocative illustration of the possibilities. As early as 1975 the scientific literature included intriguing but poorly documented claims of prolonged life in individuals with unusually high levels of HDL, a cholesterol compound that appears to operate as a scavenger to remove the residue of other cholesterol compounds from the blood. High levels of HDL or "good" cholesterol are believed to have a beneficial effect in preventing coronary heart disease. In 1990, Japanese and Columbia University researchers documented a specific defective recessive gene in five families. Individuals with two copies of the gene were unable to synthesize a protein that regulates HDL levels in the bloodstream. As a result their HDL levels were three to four times normal. Since most recessive genetic defects typically lead to premature death when the individual inherits two copies, researchers were understandably excited to observe that one of the first subjects studied had reached age 100, and had relatives who had lived well into their 80s. However, when the study was extended to five families, only two were observed to have "a trend toward longevity," and the authors conceded their evidence was purely anecdotal. That is usually a fatal flaw when it comes to the study of longevity, but the project does suggest a model for more realistic possibilities in the future.

While single-gene defects have been the initial focus of genetic research, the greatest payoff may be achieved from understanding traits influenced by several genes that interact with each other as well as the environment. Candidates for so-called polygenic traits include various cancers, obesity, many forms of heart disease, forms of high blood pressure, schizophrenia, manic-depression and a form of alcoholism. Multiple interacting genes likely also explain positive inherited traits, such as exceptional intelligence, musical and athletic ability.

Most of the scientific evidence for polygenic traits is of quite a different character from studies of the single-gene defects and is less certain. Most findings come from examining several generations of a family to measure the extent to which certain characteristics occur in a mathematical pattern suggesting a genetic inheritance. This is a more sophisticated version of the same process of systematic study through which Gregor Mendel deduced the effects of dominant and recessive traits in plants more than a century before DNA was discovered. However, this kind of statistical analysis has some of the same limitations of epidemiological studies of risk factors. Rather than providing complete evidence of a causal relationship, such analysis identifies a series of individuals who may be studied to see how their genes differ from a more typical population. Also, even when clear evidence of inherited genetic vulnerability is confirmed, it may explain only a fraction of the occurrences of the disorder.

A simple model of inherited predisposition is found in a rare eye cancer of infants and children called retinoblastoma. It affects precursor cells that mature to form the cones of the retina. A gene on chromosome 13 regulates the growth of these cells. Should both copies of the regulator gene be destroyed, the affected cell will multiply uncontrollably. Some individuals inherit one defective gene and one normal one. The tumor will result should the second gene be damaged by environmental factors or if the defective gene is copied to the normal gene by crossover during cell division. Eye tumors occur so frequently among carriers that the gene was long believed to be dominant—a single copy could cause the disease. However, at least 80 percent of all such eye tumors are not inherited. They occur among individuals with two normal copies of the gene, but in whom both copies are damaged in one of the immature retinal cells.

Another case of inherited predisposition occurs in colon cancer. Some individuals inherit the disposition to develop polyps in the intestine, and sometimes these polyps mutate into full-blown colon cancer. But again most individuals develop polyps without the gene, and polyps do not inevitably become cancers. At this writing, 1 to 2 percent of all cancers result from inherited predisposition. Cancer-causing genes, whether inherited or created through mutation, have been implicated in 10 to 15 percent of tumors. Cancer cells are not simply rogues with a simple genetic error that allows uncontrolled reproduction. Most are hardy, sophisticated survivors who have successfully evolved and multiplied in the hostile environment of a human body that is loaded with systems intended to prevent such independent action.

Much less is known about the genes that might predispose individuals toward alcoholism, obesity, schizophrenia and most forms of cancer and heart disease. As such genes are identified—and therefore can be identified in fetal DNA—society will increasingly have to wrestle with a new class of specific knowledge about individuals and their genetic advantages and disadvantages.

From advance knowledge of our genetic predispositions, it is possible to imagine great future benefits and threats that may shake the bedrock concepts of social equality in Western democracies. To know which individuals are most vulnerable to alcoholism, coronary heart disease or obesity would immediately make preventive programs enormously more effective. One important weakness of the risk factor approach to coronary heart disease, for example, is that most of those treated will never get the disease at all. Preliminary studies suggest that smoking may be enormously more hazardous to some individuals than others. To be equipped with a map of genetic strengths and weaknesses could allow someone to proceed with life in a vastly more intelligent and directed manner. It might allow society to identify and develop great potential musical, athletic or intellectual talents more effectively and provide early warning of hazards. However, the effects of more detailed genetic knowledge are not entirely positive.

Societies that cherish the notion of the equal potential of all persons must somehow come to terms with a new kind of inequality—a growing list of specific genetic advantages and disadvantages that can be measured in adults and before birth. Should airlines be allowed to reject pilots with a genetic predisposition to a premature heart attack? If it becomes possible to identify those with a strong predisposition to early-onset alcoholism, a whole new set of legal problems would immediately arise. Should such individuals be allowed to buy alcohol on the same terms as other individuals to whom it would not be so harmful? Can we hold such persons to the same standard of legal responsibility for acts committed while intoxicated?

These kinds of questions are no longer theoretical. Consider the unresolved problems created by identification of the recessive gene that causes cystic fibrosis. Should we screen all adults so the 4 percent who carry the gene can learn of the hazard to future offspring? Should couples planning to get married determine whether they are contemplating a game of genetic roulette for their children? Soon after conception, the fetuses of such couples can be tested to determine whether they carry none, one or two copies of the gene. Are parents entitled to choose to bear a child carrying two copies of the defective gene, even though it typically means death in the third decade of life after an agonizing and very expensive illness, with the medical costs paid by society? Is it anyone's right to interfere in the randomly driven genetic engine of nature through which all new human potential has developed, sometimes in new and unexpected ways? It now seems clear that the explosion of scientific knowledge about the human genome opens the door to a whole new series of difficult choices, not all of which will be welcome or easily made.

CHAPTER TWELVE

LONGEVITY ADVANTAGES

Those who are married tend to live longer than those who are divorced. College graduates have notably lower mortality rates than those who didn't finish high school. In both the United States and Europe, white-collar professionals have longer average lifespans than those with lower-skilled jobs, and the longevity differences between social classes are widening. The devout apparently enjoy measurable benefits of faith on earth as well as hereafter; Baptist ministers, Mormons and Seventh-Day Adventists, for example, have mortality rates substantially lower than the comparable general population.

What are the reasons for these longevity advantages, confirmed in repeated studies? Do marriage, a rewarding job and a good education have properties that somehow improve health status in themselves? Or are those individuals simply healthier and more vigorous than others? Do we best understand longevity by viewing humans as biological machines playing out a series of programmed genetic instructions in a particular environment, harsh or gentle? Or do the social interactions of marriage, job and community play as important a role as individual health factors such as diabetes and blood pressure?

The central themes of this book hold that all the above propositions are true. Not only are the factors that influence health and longevity incredibly diverse, they interact to produce magnified effects, both positive and negative. Alcohol abuse, for example, is independently associated with an elevated death rate from liver damage, violence, suicide and heart disease. However, alcohol abuse is simultaneously a possible cause and frequently observed effect of a failed marriage. And one expects alcohol abuse to be less common among the strictly religious. To appreciate the interplay of health behaviors, disease, psychosocial factors and the environment is to embrace, in all its rich breadth and depth, a world of longevity in which the whole is vastly larger than the sum of its parts.

Examining a larger universe of influences on longevity helps explain why trying to achieve small changes in narrowly defined risk factors produces such disappointing results. The history of scientific achievement instructs us that most discoveries about man and nature have come through breaking down complex processes and mastering the laws governing the most rudimentary component parts. However, this time-tested reductionist approach has been less successful in explaining differences in human longevity. We are each so different, with our own unique selection of genes, living in different environments that may variously protect and harm us. And perhaps the most intriguing component of our environment is the ways that humans nurture and harm each other. As might be expected, one of the greatest of these influences is wielded by the person with whom we are most intimate, a spouse.

The institution of marriage, therefore, makes a good beginning point for the examination of longevity advantages. In modern Western societies, more than 9 out of 10 adults marry at least once; among American adults, slightly less than one-quarter are single at any particular point in time. Numerous studies rate the dissolution of marriage by death, divorce or separation as the most stressful event in a lifetime. It outranks a contemplated jail term, dismissal from job, difficulties with sex or retirement as the most stressful and requiring the most far-reaching adjustments. Not surprisingly, excess mortality has also been repeatedly observed among the unmarried, widowed, divorced and separated. It was identified among members of the European nobility in the fifteenth century, and confirmed in an 1848 study of French society. Modern studies embracing the United States, western Europe and Japan show the pattern of excess mortality among the unmarried is universal among the advanced, long-lived societies.

Another important trend can be identified across a wide variety of modern cultures. Measured by mortality, women benefit from marriage less than men. They also report lower rates of satisfaction with being married. Conversely, whether they never married or were widowed, separated or divorced, women fared better than men when single. In a few societies, notably Japan, the highest excess mortality rates were found among men who never married. In most other countries, the largest number of excess deaths occur among divorced, widowed and separated men.

A federal Mortality Study of One Million persons showed 45 percent excess mortality among divorced white males, and 23 percent among divorced white women. The male excess mortality is roughly comparable with the risks reported earlier for mild high blood pressure and severe obesity. In the case of severed marriages, however, the excess risks declined with advancing age, leaving a paradox. At younger ages when overall mortality rates are lowest, the effect of divorce and separation was largest. An American study confined to individuals under age 65, for example, found divorced men with mortality rates 340 percent higher than married men. For younger women, death rates were 200 percent higher. A 1992 study showed that men who survived one heart attack were twice as likely to die of a second event in the next six months if they lived alone rather than with a spouse. However, as overall death rates rise with advancing age, the effect of divorce, separation and being a widow become increasingly overshadowed by rising mortality from all causes.

Do we suppose, however, that the divorced and separated are identical with married persons except for their marital status? Or does selection bias occur? In other words, are divorced men vulnerable in other ways, so that marriage amounts to something like the healthy worker effect observed in the introductory chapter, selecting the healthiest and more vigorous? A study of young and middle-aged men in Gothenburg, Sweden, provides some intriguing insights. In all, death rates were 260 percent higher among divorced men, when compared with the married men. Marital status, however, was only one of many differences. For example, 26 percent of the divorced men had been treated for alcohol abuse, compared with 5 percent of the married men. Among the divorced men, 11 percent were receiving economic assistance, compared with 4 percent of the married men. The divorced men were also more likely to be smokers, to report being under severe stress and to have lower-skilled occupations. Therefore, divorce also describes a group of men with an entire portfolio of influences associated with higher mortality rates.

In this instance, the science of statistics rides partly to the rescue. All these influences can be separated statistically, and the effect of divorce measured after adjusting for the other known influences on mortality. In this case, the other factors accounted for one-third of the excess mortality. The remaining two-thirds appeared to be the result of marital status. But, unfortunately, real life is not as tidy as mathematics. As noted, other studies reveal that men are more likely to drink and smoke when divorced than when married. Should we consider smoking and drinking an entirely separate "health behavior" issue—or partly a consequence of divorce? It also works the other way. Men who abuse alcohol are more likely to become divorced in the first place. So perhaps alcohol abuse as readily damages marriages as it does health.

How does one sort out these diverse and interacting influences? While marriage apparently does have inherent value to health, it is also an important marker for successful biological and social adjustment. And those who make the most successful adjustments to the pressures and demands of life will live the longest. So diverse are the reasons for failure to adjust that it is more appropriate to observe simply that marriage is an important indicator of success. There are, however, equally revealing psychosocial markers.

While money may not buy happiness, higher income and higher social/economic status are unmistakably associated with a longer lifespan. One perspective comes from the government's Mortality Study of One Million. Up to age 65, death rates in the poorest families (those earning $8,000 a year or less) were 250 percent higher than families prosperous enough to earn $65,000, or about twice the typical American family's income. Such differences in death rates for social class or income category have been observed in the United States and Europe for 150 years.

The rich and poor nevertheless die of roughly the same causes. In rank order, the leading modern killers remain heart disease, cancer, and the nonmedical causes accidents, suicide and homicide. In Third World nations—or the advanced nations of a century ago—an entirely different pattern of mortality prevails, featuring high infant and childhood mortality and large numbers of premature deaths from infectious disease.

Among the modern poor, the main causes of death resemble those of the most prosperous, but the poor die of heart disease, cancer and external causes at rates that are two and a half times higher. The same pattern could be found among the English in 1850. The prosperous and well-fed aristocracy suffered from the same basic hazards as the poor of the time: large losses of infants and children, and high death rates from tuberculosis and pneumonia. The lesson of these similarities and differences is this: The rich and poor, privileged and disadvantaged, nevertheless share the common perils of a particular time and place. But for reasons worth exploring further, the advantaged seem to enjoy a better overall health status. This is quite a different pattern than if we discovered that money could somehow purchase immunity from some major cause of death that still devastated the poor.

Longevity benefits have been systematically observed for other measures of social/economic advantage or social class. The Mortality Study of One Million showed that among those who didn't finish high school, death rates were 95 percent higher than for those who completed college. This difference was in premature deaths occurring in adult males before age 64; once again the contrasts were smaller among the elderly. In the United States death rates also vary among occupations, with mortality rates lowest among professional and technical workers, and highest among laborers.

It seems certain that high-level education, occupation and income are separate measures that describe a similar population of individuals with life expectancy advantages. While there are other factors of some importance, all are measures of successful adjustment to the current demands of modern society. Those who complete 16 years of education, and obtain a professional job with good pay are a population with above-average intelligence, without crippling health problems, and with average or better social skills. Not only was this group blessed by some inherent biological advantages, they applied these skills with reasonable levels of effort. Thus the longevity advantages flow to individuals capable of prospering within the confining but substantial demands of the modern technical society. The figures above were for white males; the differences are smaller for women. Most studies are not large enough to provide accurate data for blacks or other minorities.

In England, the United States, Denmark and Sweden, this longevity gap defined by social and economic status has apparently increased over recent decades. This seemingly ominous trend, however, supports conflicting interpretations. One might argue this demonstrates that social inequality must be growing because the socially and economically advantaged increasingly exploit those less fortunate. However, if these societies were increasingly successful in providing equal opportunities for education and employment, the observed result would be exactly the same. If the best education and jobs increasingly went to the most able and vigorous—rather than to an arbitrarily selected group with inherited advantages—the longevity gap would still be expected to widen.

It is also possible those with more education and ability are taking conscious steps to prolong their lives, taking actions seen less frequently among those with less education, lower intelligence, or less-skilled jobs. Increased rates of smoking, alcohol abuse, drug abuse and obesity have all been observed among those with low social/economic status. The evidence for a behavioral factor is strongest for smoking, which has declined rapidly among those with college education. The Mortality Study of One Million contained a special section analyzing the effect of smoking. It showed, for example, that only 15 percent of those with postcollege education smoked, compared with 45 percent of those who didn't complete high school. As a second step the author, epidemiologist Eugene Rogot, adjusted the figures for the likely mortality effects of smoking. Rogot's analysis showed lower incidence of smoking was one factor, but it accounted for only a small part of the mortality advantages observed for those with more education, better occupation and higher income.

The most ambitious attempt to separate risk factors and health behaviors from social and economic advance occurred in the Gothenburg, Sweden, study cited earlier on the effects of marital status. It divided a study population of 7,000 middle-aged men into four occupational classes. Unskilled and semiskilled workers were the lowest class, and executives, professionals and high-level civil servants in the highest. Overall differences in mortality rates were similar to those observed in the United States. The mortality rate in the lowest occupational class was 2.1 times higher than in the highest. Then the investigators adjusted for all the differences that could be explained by the following factors: smoking, treatment for alcohol abuse, being overweight, cholesterol level, blood pressure, leisure time, physical activity, marital status, diabetes and family history of heart disease. Taken altogether these factors accounted for almost half the difference—but the effect of occupational class remained an important factor. As noted with marital status, these mathematical techniques do not measure the likely interactions among these factors. But such analysis does make remote the possibility that occupational and class differences are simply an artifact of other underlying factors.

Not only are social, economic or occupational advantages associated with longer lifespans, they also have impressive predictive powers. The most dramatic demonstration of this can be found in a study of 85,500 military veterans discharged in 1946, just after the close of World War II. The enormous numbers of individuals drafted, trained and dispatched around the world had a disruptive effect on the normal operations of social and economic class.

Here is how the death rates compared over the 23 years after discharge from the military:

Rank	Mortality Rates Compared with General Population
Officers	59%
Noncommissioned officers	77%
Privates	100%

Simultaneously one can also observe the effects of educational attainment:

MORTALITY RATE COMPARED WITH GENERAL POPULATION		
Education	Officers	Privates
Grammar school	89%	101%
High school	55%	77%
College	49%	81%

As in the other studies, the privates tended to die of the same causes as the longer-lived officers, but at consistently higher rates. The military operates as a rigid class system. But the differences in life expectancy were observed after discharge during an expansionary economic period that offered hitherto unprecedented economic mobility and opportunity. And to enter wartime military service, the entire group had to be free of any important impairments to health. While once again, several factors contributed, it seems likely that the officers were a group with above-average health, vigor and intelligence, and therefore less vulnerable to death from all causes.

Such studies raise profound questions about social equality and the equality of opportunity. A provocative test of one's perceptions is to guess the long-term longevity effects on a group of individuals with an abrupt change in one of the three indicators—income, occupation or education—but not the others. What would happen to a group of well-educated professionals who were suddenly plunged into poverty in a strange land—the real-life situation of some immigrants. After 20 years would their life expectancy resemble that of other low-income families, or those with similar education or occupational status? Or what would be the effects of offering free education to individuals who failed to graduate from high school? The real-life counterpart can be found in numerous high-school equivalency and job training programs—an intentional effort to use education to improve an individual's social status, occupation and income. Since there are no data on this question, the answers are left to the reader.

Important longevity advantages have also been observed repeatedly among the devout. A careful study of Baptist ministers, for example, revealed their chances of dying prematurely were only 56 percent of a comparable population of white males. Similar advantages were observed among Lutheran, Presbyterian and Episcopal ministers. However, one immediately suspects selection bias, since these life expectancy advantages are quite similar to those cited earlier for veterans who served as officers and for college-educated professionals. Also, the causes of death were once again quite similar to the general population—just occurring at lower rates.

A more provocative contrast is the increased longevity observed among Mormons and Seventh-Day Adventists in California. Both religions proscribe smoking, and the effect on lung cancer death rates in men is dramatic—only 18 percent of the death rate in a comparable general population. Among female Seventh-Day Adventists the lung cancer death rate is 33 percent of a comparable general population. This is one of the largest differences in cause-specific mortality in the scientific literature. And this is cause-specific gain. Unlike previous examples which primarily involved identifying a population with a more robust overall health status, the Mormons and Seventh-Day Adventists appear to enjoy specific health benefits of a particular practice—refraining from smoking.

But lower lung cancer rates—and even the effects of having so few smokers—do not fully explain the longevity advantages enjoyed by these two groups. The overall risk of premature death among adult males who were California Mormon and Seventh-Day Adventists was approximately 50 percent of the general population. As in all of these psychosocial measures, the differences were smaller among women, and became less important with increasing age. At least three factors were involved in the increased life expectancy observed in these groups. Selection bias still operates because members of these religions are better educated, have higher-than-average incomes, and are more likely to be married and have professional jobs. Second is the effect of not smoking and possible effects of the proscription of alcohol. Finally there are likely psychosocial benefits from belonging to a tight-knit social group with shared values and rules for living. It would not be surprising to observe lower mortality rates among tight-knit religious groups whether they prescribed particular health behaviors or not.

An unresolved question surrounds one aspect of the Seventh-Day Adventists' lifestyle. The church recommends (but does not demand) that members refrain from eating meat, poultry or beef, and these dietary guidelines are followed by roughly one-half of its members. (Dairy products and eggs, however, are allowed.) It is claimed that this may account for the lower rates of heart disease observed among its members. The Seventh-Day Adventist studies are simply not well enough controlled to judge one way or another. Because it is the leading cause of death, coronary heart disease deaths are reduced in virtually any population with lower mortality rates. Only some church members follow the diet, and have adhered to the guidelines for varying periods of time. A properly controlled study would examine two groups that differ only in dietary practices, and address the possibility that a vegetarian diet might lower mortality rates from coronary heart disease but raise them for other causes, perhaps stomach cancer and stroke.

. . .

Many people suppose that better medical care explains the longer lifespans among the better educated and more prosperous. The available evidence, however, suggests this is probably not the case. If the primary missing element were medical care, then we should expect to find the excess deaths concentrated among ailments where medical care is dramatically effective—for example, pneumonia, syphilis and other controllable infectious diseases, diabetes, intestinal obstructions and kidney failure. Instead we find most deaths occurring among the same major causes where medical interventions are not so effective: accidents, violence, suicide, cancer and heart disease.

Perhaps even more compelling is the fact that those with lower social and economic status consistently consume more medical care than the more prosperous—primarily because their health status is generally worse. The federal Health Interview Survey, for example, shows the poor are more likely than nonpoor to be in fair or poor health, to have a disabling condition, to need hospital care, to contact a physician and to require medical attention for injury from accidents or violence.

Also, in most Western societies medical care is distributed vastly more equitably than either income or education. The United States still does not have universal health insurance, consigning roughly 30 million lower-income but employed individuals to receive only emergency medical care. And excess deaths preventable by medical treatment unquestionably occur in the most-deprived populations. But this cannot account for but a fraction of the broad mortality trend observed throughout the social and economic spectrum. As social and economic status falls, mortality rates rise. What forces could underlie this increased vulnerability to damage from many causes?

Those who achieve more successful biological and social adaptation are experiencing lower long-term levels of stress. Unfortunately, the term *stress* is one of those words that everybody knows but that actually describes several different kinds of problems. Stress, in the engineering sense, means an increased burden on some system. Both high blood pressure and running a mile place stress on the circulatory system. Extreme cold places extra stress on body metabolism, while extreme heat makes other demands. Consuming large amounts of salt—or abstaining entirely—places unusual demands on the series of hormones that regulate the concentration of sodium and potassium in the blood. Similar biological stresses can be created in response to consuming large quantities of alcohol. As was observed earlier in obesity, a disorder that begins as a biological regulation problem may end up creating obstacles to social interactions. Or as with some forms of alcoholism, a problem that may originate in social interactions ultimately has a direct biological consequence—cirrhosis of the liver. It is easily shown that negative social inputs can create biological disorders.

It is likely, but certainly less well established, that positive social interactions elicit better performance from biological systems. Not only do social and biological systems interact, but another important characteristic of stress is apparent from these examples. The body is designed to adjust to such stresses occasionally, and may benefit directly from experiencing periods of stress. This certainly is the logic behind exercise, steam rooms and skydiving. The damaging stresses are the excessive demands on the system that are constant and unrelenting.

When discussing stress, many people mean something else entirely. They mean psychological stress rather than the narrower biological kind. Examined carefully, what people normally mean by psychological stress is a specific kind of biological stress. Faced with situations that trigger the emotions of anxiety, excitement, anger or fear, the body is flooded with a casade of hormones intended to enhance its capacity to fight or flee. Some individuals crave this hormonal hit, among them performers, athletes, mountain climbers and sky divers. As with other kinds of biological stress, the damage occurs when such signals are received constantly—such as among paramedics or police officers patrolling areas with high levels of violence. Some studies have found that on-the-job stresses are most harmful when the individual has little latitude to respond to the hormonal alarm signals, for example, among telephone solicitors or assembly-line workers. It seems evident that a permanent state of poverty, where individuals cannot obtain the essentials of adequate food, clothing, safety and shelter must also must create the destructive kind of recurring stress.

The central theme of this book—that the longest lifespans will be observed among those who adapt most successfully—suggests that stress is not harmful in itself. Stress is a term that describes the signals that the biological and social systems send to demand action—or to enable an individual to take action to adjust to a specific environment. It seems obvious that individuals who are receiving constant biological stress signals from their marriage or job may not need to better tolerate the distress signals—so-called stress management. They should change the conditions that are causing these distress signals to be sent. That, simply put, is the beginning of the process of successful adaptation. Stress is the signal that action is required.

No one would suggest the game of successful adaptation takes place on a level playing field. As was seen in the chapter on obesity, some individuals must undertake a lifelong regimen of food monitoring and restraint simply to equal the effortless weight regulation that many others enjoy automatically. Some individuals unconsciously regulate their alcohol intake, while others must build elaborate systems of social support to achieve abstinence. The interactions between divorce, alcohol and smoking also suggest that failure feeds on itself. Similarly, the reinforcing effects of achievement in education, occupation and income suggest that each successful adaptation brings the next problem closer to solution. This helps explain why once individuals begin to acquire a few longevity advantages, they are likely to end up with a generous supply of them.

3

THE SCIENCE OF LONGEVITY

CHAPTER THIRTEEN

THE LIFESPAN OF CELLS
AND OTHER CREATURES

Why can't a man be more like a worm? If humans shared more common biology with the ubiquitous, unsegmented worms called nematodes, the genetic tools to extend our maximum lifespan might soon be within the grasp of science. In a University of Colorado microbiology laboratory, Thomas E. Johnson has isolated a single mutation of a gene that he calls *age-1*. Garden-variety soil nematodes, carrying a normal version of *age-1,* live a maximum of 37 days in Johnson's lab.

Nematodes are observably subject to a central law of biology that operates in similar fashion in humans. It is called the force of mortality, or Gompertz's law, and was formulated in 1825 by an English mathematician of the same name. It holds that after reaching maturity, the mortality rate of most animal species rises in exponential fashion, at first a slow upward rise, then later sweeping irresistibly upward toward a certain and finite end. In soil nematodes, the mortality rate doubles every 3.5 days; in humans roughly every 8 years. This relentless doubling of mortality rates produces a maximum lifespan, a theoretical point where there should be no survivors of even a very large population. This remains a fixed limit even if premature deaths are reduced.

Many observers believe that major increases in human longevity will be achieved through altering the central underlying force of mortality rather than by the current strategy of separately attacking the myriad disorders of advancing age. It is therefore of great interest that Johnson appears to have successfully modified one of the great immutable laws of biology, shifting the entire mortality curve.

The nematodes that carry two copies of the mutant *age-1* gene have maximum lifespans that are twice as long as their more ordinary cousins. The relentless upward Gompertzian march of the mortality rate was altered. Instead of doubling every 3.5 days, mortality rates took more than 7 days to double. This feat, measured on a human time scale, would mean achieving an average lifespan of 130 years in scores of individuals, with some surviving to a maximum age of 230 years. The long-lived nematodes had a normal life cycle of growth and reproduction, and demonstrated an increased maximum lifespan under varying environmental conditions. However, other than being confident of the existence of a genuine longevity gene, researchers do not know what biological function *age-1* actually performs.

Johnson's and other experiments with nematode genes are exciting not because they are soon likely to usher in similar control over the human lifespan. Nematodes are extraordinarily simple creatures with about 1 percent the number of genes in humans; since they are hermaphrodites, the presence of both male and female sexual organs makes inbreeding simple. And it should be remembered that doubling a nematode's maximum lifespan is still an increase of about a month.

Nevertheless, it remains a breathtaking achievement. Humans have actually grasped new genetic controls of this great machine of life hurtling through space and time. To tinker with the very structure of mortality itself seems a dizzying power, an act almost as audacious as trying to alter gravity or the flow of time. For many decades humans have been successful in altering the average lifespan or life expectancy. But in humans, the maximum lifespan, guarded by the relentless upsweep of mortality rates, has thus far remained a final, unassailable barrier.

In humans, that barrier apparently is at 115 years of age. Highly publicized claims have been made for unusual longevity among residents in the Caucasus Mountains of Georgia and in the mountains of Kashmir and the Andes. Such claims, however, are not supported by valid birth records or other supporting documents. They are based on much more fallible human memories. In one such community, Vilcabamba in the Andes Mountains of Ecuador, there is no written language, let alone records. Investigators who visited Vilcabamba after a five-year absence, discovered that the subjects claimed ages that were seven to ten years older than during the previous visit. Zhores Medvedev, the Russian geneticist and longevity researcher, found a curious trend in the Caucasus. The earlier in this century that literacy and record keeping were introduced, the fewer the claims of unusually long life. In short, when dependable written records replace more fallible memories, claims of unusually long life disappear.

Although 115 years is the standard figure cited in most of the aging literature, some papers on this question argue no good proof exists for anyone surviving past age 110. The difference between the two estimates is probably not of great significance. The underlying arithmetic of rising mortality rates predicts that there should be no survivors past 115 years even in a very large population. Even if an exception were discovered, it would not affect the implications of the mortality curve. To rewrite these laws of mortality would require a large number of exceptions.

So high are mortality rates late in life that the chances of reaching even age 100 are quite small, even with modern-era life expectancies approaching age 80. Among 100,000 males, just 368 will reach age 100 at current mortality rates, and only 1 lives to age 110. And nobody survives to 116. Although long-term evidence is almost entirely lacking, there is no reason to suppose that the maximum lifespan has changed over many centuries.

However, a lifespan of fixed maximum length is no accident of nature, nor is it an invariable by-product of some physical law such as momentum or friction. The truth of this proposition can be readily observed in the animal kingdom. The most imaginative and detailed analysis comes from a University of Chicago neurobiologist named Caleb E. Finch. The maximum lifespan of the familiar household mouse is 4 to 5 years. However, another small mammal of similar size, the brown bat, can live at least 32 years. Why does one small mammal live seven times longer than another? Is the maximum lifespan under control of a relatively simple genetic clock? This possibility is suggested by the comparison of humans with our closest animal relative, the chimpanzee. Given that 95 percent of the genes are identical in both animals, why is there no record of a chimpanzee surviving more than 44 years, when the human maximum is apparently 115 years? While the difference between the two primate species is likely to be more complex than the *age-1* gene in nematodes, the comparison does hint at the existence of a relatively small number of human longevity genes.

When small rodents succumb to exponentially rising mortality rates after two or three years, they die of many different specific ailments, just as humans do after many decades of life. Not only is the pattern similar, so are many of the specific disorders. With advancing age rats stop reproducing; they gain weight; key hormone levels fall; they get diabetes and arthritis, suffer kidney failure, and most notably, die of cancer. Why is this chaotic pattern of decay, called biological senescence, observed over such different intervals of time? The relationship of cancer and aging is particularly provocative. Cancer is apparently initiated by sunlight, radiation, environmental toxins, viruses and possibly other factors that damage the genes controlling cell reproduction. This conjures up an image of inevitable but random damage to DNA, which ultimately suffers a hit on a critical segment of the genetic code. But why is this damage so widespread in 27-month-old laboratory mice, but extremely rare in 27-month-old humans? This strongly suggests the presence of a reasonably effective defense against this threat or the ability to repair its damage. Is this capacity deliberately turned off at different times in species with varying lifespans?

Researchers probing the frontiers of longevity have sometimes moved well beyond the ability to pose interesting questions and assemble tantalizing clues. As this is written, at least three substances with antiaging properties in animals are being tested in humans with federal research funds. One of them is human growth hormone, another is a steroid hormone of mysterious purpose known as DHEA, and the third is a family of chemicals called antioxidants; vitamin C is the best-known example. Researchers routinely take human cell cultures with a fixed lifespan and make them immortal and, at will, restore immortal cells to the normal process of deterioration with increasing age. Thus far, the unfortunate tradeoff is that the immortal cells are cancer cells. Using diet, researchers can alter the average and the maximum lifespan of several small mammals, as well as much simpler creatures such as rotifers and nematodes.

The science of longevity, however, remains in its infancy. It is characterized by a diverse collection of exciting but often utterly conflicting ideas. Numerous theories flower only when no imposing body of empirical fact intrudes to hinder the limitless human imagination: Do the same hormonal changes that bring sexual maturity also trigger other processes that ultimately ensure death? Does a master clock time all four major stages of life—gestation, development, maturity and decline—and can this clock be reset? Or is aging an irregular process of cumulative damage at the cellular level, leaving most cells battered but functional until some catastrophic error occurs?

Enormous gaps exist in our knowledge of fundamentals essential to serious and sustained progress and to test most theories. For example, suppose that one of the substances now being tested in humans does have important antiaging properties. How would we ever know? Beyond the crude and cumbersome chronological age, no consistent method exists to measure whether an underlying process of aging is being retarded or accelerated. In one project, 28 different markers of human aging were identified. None were satisfactory, and few were consistent with each other. The National Institute on Aging is spending $30 million on a ten-year project to develop reliable biomarkers in rats, whose lifespan can be manipulated. In the meantime, however, researchers will have to use stopgap alternatives which are not entirely satisfactory. For example, it is feasible to study the shortest-lived rodents, whose total lifespan can be observed and measured. But will anything be learned about the longest-lived animals by focusing on the shortest-lived animals? We might find drugs capable of preventing certain cancers, reversing the loss of muscle mass, or repairing other individual indicators of age such as wrinkled and spotted skin. But without better biomarkers of aging, there would be little assurance that widespread use of these drugs would lengthen life rather than shorten it. Even if the study of aging is confined to the most elemental cellular level, scores of different changes have been identified, without clues to which are the important ones. Given the mysteries remaining at the cellular level, what are the prospects for the effects of aging in complex animals with trillions of interacting cells?

The promising clues combined with great uncertainties are what make longevity the most exciting little backwater of science. Understanding the underlying process of aging may ultimately mean identifying common factors in cancer, heart disease, arthritis, osteoporosis, non-insulin-dependent diabetes, hypertension, Alzheimer's disease, kidney disease and other disorders. But in the world of biomedical research, aging is very much the neglected child. In the United States, for example, the National Institutes of Health spend $1.5 billion annually for cancer research, $1 billion annually for heart disease research and nearly

$100 billion annually for treatment of these two degenerative diseases. A tiny fraction of that sum, less than $100 million, is spent on aging research. Thus, for every one thousand dollars spent on coronary heart disease and cancer, less than a dollar goes to understand the basic process that may underlie both disorders. Even the agency responsible for this research area, the National Institute on Aging, does not rate research on the aging process as its most important task. Research on a specific disease, Alzheimer's, is its current top priority.

"No congressman's relatives or constituents ever die of basic biology," said NIA associate director Richard Sprott. "The way the government science game is being played these days, Congress is specifically funding certain kinds of issues." He noted that Congress was responding to public concerns, fueled in part by an energetic citizens' organization that had successfully built a grass-roots constituency demanding more research on Alzheimer's. But Sprott, who heads both Alzheimer's and basic aging research at NIA, believes the breakthroughs will come from more basic understanding of the aging process.

"I believe that ultimately the solution to most of the problems we're talking about is going to come from basic biological research, and not from research on how to treat the symptoms of diseases that already exist," he said. However, the baffling nature of the aging process and the modest resources invested mean that these exciting possibilities are unlikely to produce practical benefits in the immediate future.

Nature instructs us that many methods exist to terminate the lives of cells, body parts and entire organisms that have outlived their usefulness. Each of us once had webbed feet and hands. But before birth, the appropriate cells obediently died on command, at a particular time set on the gestational clock. These changes are small in comparison with the spectacular cell death and transfiguration that occur when a pupa becomes a butterfly.

In some species, the lifespan of entire organisms is regulated with the same iron-fisted genetic control. Honeybees are a dramatic example. The same fertilized egg can produce creatures with three different finite lifespans. The worker bees that are hatched during the warm months of the year live one or two months. However, if they hatch during the winter they may survive up to one year. If "royal jelly" is added to the egg, however, the result is a queen bee with a typical lifespan of five years. She makes a single mating flight, receiving sperm from a sequence of drones. When her store of sperm is depleted, she is killed by the workers. In some social insects, the queen survives up to 15 years; in others, her lifespan is similar to that of the workers. Short-lived workers, long-lived workers and queens have the same genes.

In other animals, a fixed lifespan is deeply embedded in the very architecture of their plan of life. An extreme example is the mayfly, which lives only a few hours after hatching. It has no mouth or digestive system and dies as soon as its inborn stores of energy are exhausted. Its sole adult function is to mate. The bamboo plant can live for a century, but it dies as soon as it flowers. Grazing mammals die when their teeth wear out, one of the cases where lifespan is limited by mechanical wear and tear. But since some mammals—rats, for example—have continuously growing teeth, this leaves unresolved the question of whether grazing animals are a case of genetic design or mechanical failure.

In the life plan of some animal species, death is an immediate by-product of one-time reproduction. The salmon executes a frenzied journey up the freshwater stream of its birth, reproduces, and then dies. In some species of lamprey, a primitive predecessor of fish, the animal literally melts away after spawning. It stops eating; the intestine deteriorates, the liver shrinks; body stores of fat and protein are consumed. In one species of Australian marsupial mice, the males die at one year of age from the stress of a 12-hour sexual orgy of repeated copulation. If captured and isolated before breeding, they live two or three times as long.

While only in rare instances do humans die as a direct consequence of reproduction, longevity researchers have observed one striking and possibly applicable fact about many of these animals. A specific hormonal trigger causes the sequence of one-time reproduction and death. If the hormonal trigger is disabled, the animal neither reproduces nor dies immediately. In humans the cessation of growth, the maturation of sexual organs, and other physical developments are the result of hormonal changes. Perhaps this is how the human lifespan is also regulated. It is also no coincidence that two of the three substances that may have antiaging properties in humans are hormones.

Some animals appear to have no fixed lifespan, and do not experience the myriad indications of decay with aging. Barnacles, lobsters, turtles, rockfish and sturgeon appear to have escaped the exponential increase in mortality rates observed in most other animals. These animals are not immortal—a fraction of their number die each year. But they may have no fixed outer limit. According to a tabulation prepared by Alex Comfort, an important British longevity researcher, a species of turtle called Marian's tortoise has lived 158 years, longer than any mammal, including humans. Several Carolina box tortoises have lived more than 120 years. An 85-year-old sturgeon has been caught in the United States. And 40-pound lobsters have been found, suggesting a lifespan of 50 to 100 years.

Animals without a fixed maximum lifespan share several important characteristics. Unlike mammals, they do not grow to a fixed size. Both growth and life continue indefinitely. These animals also remain fertile throughout life, while reproduction ceases in mammals once the fixed supply of eggs has been exhausted. Also, none are warm-blooded. Animals with indefinite lifespans are the exceptions that seem to establish a rule: If such huge variations in lifespan and life plan are found, then it seems unlikely that some unalterable biochemical factor underlies the aging process. However, virtually all case studies from the animal kingdom are subject to great uncertainty. Those described above are accepted by major authorities in the field—for example, Comfort and Caleb Finch. But both authors note the tremendous difficulties in determining average and maximum lifespans. In captivity, lifespans can be observed precisely, but it is likely the artificial conditions of captivity shorten life. Animals might, in theory, live longer in the wild. But losses to predators, disease and accidents are so great that few ever approach the biological maximum—whatever it might be.

The two extreme life strategies—tightly programmed rapid death and an indefinite lifespan—help define the middle ground occupied by humans, all mammals and most warm-blooded animals. Like those species where death seems clearly written into the genetic program, humans and other mammals have fixed maximum lifespans. In another way, however, the aging process in mammals is quite unlike that seen in the creatures who grow old and die quickly under a clear genetic mandate. In those animals the cause of aging is clear and obvious: mayflies have no means to eat, salmon are flooded with a hormone. In the final one-third of life, humans undergo so many biological changes that there is not even agreement about which constitute aging and which do not. As a life strategy, Caleb Finch calls this gradual senescence (or aging) with definite lifespan.

The confounding fact about gradual senescence is that the indications of aging vary enormously among individuals. There are changes in hair, teeth, sight, hearing, skin, body fat, muscles, hormone levels, liver, kidneys, bones, blood pressure, blood sugar, and in skeletal, reproductive, circulatory and immune systems. Nor do these changes occur uniformly even if one assumes that biological and chronological age might differ. Some people have all their hair and teeth in their 80s, and some have neither. Neither of these decrements of age likely affects the maximum lifespan. Not only do the manifestations of aging differ among individuals, they may not affect either life expectancy or the maximum lifespan.

Some longevity researchers argue that since aging is a universal process, true aging changes also must be universal. Cancer, therefore, would not be a manifestation of aging because a majority of people never get cancer, no matter how long they live. Neither would stroke or coronary heart disease be considered aging. In this view, these disorders might shorten the life of some people, but they are separate and unrelated diseases. On the other hand, menopause in women and changes in the eye lens occur universally. This might force research to focus on the fundamental underlying processes, rather than on surface manifestations, but this definition seems too narrow and confining to be useful. It's more productive to realize that a key characteristic of aging is that it is a heterogenous process with great variations among individuals. We are all put together differently, and spend our lives exposed to and protected from different hazards. It should not be so surprising that we also age differently. But this makes the measurement and possible alteration of the aging process problematical. If we can't say precisely what aging is, how will we ever know if we have slowed or halted it? These are the kinds of intellectual dilemmas that plague this infant science.

In the pursuit of greater simplicity and precision, some savvy longevity researchers have chosen to bypass these problems entirely. Instead they have focused on thousands of truly identical cells growing under completely controlled and uniform conditions in a laboratory. After all, we are a vast collection of individual cells that happen to work together. Therefore, the aging process ought to be taking place inside those cells. And one important line of evidence suggests the controls on lifespan must exist at the cellular level.

Until 1961, biologists believed there was little point in studying the aging process in cells. Individual cells were thought to be capable of living and proliferating forever if provided with the proper environment and nutrients. A pioneering longevity researcher named Leonard Hayflick demonstrated convincingly that all normal human cells were, in fact, mortal.

Hayflick experimented with a prolific and hardy human cell known as a fibroblast, which differentiates and multiplies to form soft connective tissue throughout the body. He grew fibroblasts in laboratory bottles that could be laid on their flat rectangular sides, providing an even surface where cells could anchor and grow. The fibroblasts were provided with nutrients and incubated at room temperature. In roughly one week's time, the flat side of the bottle would be covered with a uniform layer of fibroblasts exactly one cell in thickness. Then the cells would stop dividing because of contact inhibition. Next Hayflick put one half the cells in an empty bottle. They resumed dividing once again until the surface was again entirely covered with a uniform layer of cells. He could repeat this procedure 50 times. But as the cells approached their 50th population doubling, things began to change. Cell multiplication began to take longer—ten days to fill the flat surface of the bottle instead of the usual seven. And after about 50 population doublings, the cells never again filled the bottom of the bottle. They continued to live for days, but finally died of a variety of causes. This is the seminal demonstration of one fixed limit on human life. Human cell populations can double about 50 times and no more. Each individual cell, of course, did not divide exactly 50 times. Some divided more, some not at all. But they all got old and died, just like we do.

Since this experiment contradicted the existing belief that individual cells are immortal, Hayflick's discovery was received skeptically. Maybe the cells died because he got the nutrients wrong or introduced contaminants? To prove that wasn't the case, Hayflick and his colleague, Paul S. Moorhead, combined cells of two different ages. One group of male fibroblasts had doubled 40 times; the female fibroblasts just 10 times. Because of the X and Y sex chromosomes, it was possible to tell them apart under a microscope. After another 20 doublings, only the younger female fibroblasts survived. The older male counterparts had reached the limit of 50, and then died.

The demonstration of a limit on cell division has proved to be extraordinarily durable. Fibroblasts could be frozen for years with liquid nitrogen. When thawed, they resumed the cycle of doubling until reaching the limit of 50. And then they died. At warmer temperatures they multiplied faster, at cooler temperatures more slowly. But still just about 50 population doublings occurred. They got fibroblasts from both young and old adults. Adult cells of any age doubled fewer times than the embryonic cells. But the cells from younger adults did not always double more times than those of older adults, as one might expect. The reasons for this mysterious finding have never been explained. However, the overall limit of 50 population doublings is so regular that it suggests the cell must have some kind of molecular clock. How else could it determine its own age with reasonable precision?

Hayflick's discovery proved so enduring, and so readily confirmed, that it has become a central reference point for the study of aging at the cellular level. The landmark experiment also helped make Hayflick one of the grand old men of a very young science.

However, a limit on cell doubling of 50 does not, on its face, seem to limit humans to a 115-year maximum lifespan. For example, we certainly should not run short of connective tissue from the fibroblasts. One fibroblast cell, subject to 50 population doublings, grows exponentially to produce almost 500 billion pounds of cells! Also, skeletal muscle cells and nerve cells do not multiply· at all after differentiating and maturing. Yet they operate for more than a century after their last cell division. "We do not believe that aging results from a loss of cell division potential," Hayflick flatly declares.

What it does mean, Hayflick believes, is that the aging process is a direct function of the cell machinery. Loss of ability to divide is one of 200 different changes believed to occur inside a cell with increasing age. Another, for example, is the accumulation of a dark pigment called lipofuscin, which in itself is apparently harmless. Lipofuscin is most visible as liver spots in older skin, but also accumulates in other cells.

The cell division limit conceivably could be a life-lengthening evolutionary by-product: Perhaps after 50 divisions, cells are likely to have accumulated enough damage or other irregular features to make a proliferative shutdown a good bet. Nevertheless, it is one of the few precisely defined, inevitable and universal phenomena of aging. However, the experiment by no means describes the general behavior of all cells. The limit of 50 population doublings applies specifically to *normal human* cells.

Some cells are indeed immortal. Primitive bacterial cells live forever. But they have neither the nucleus nor all the elaborate specialized structures in differentiated human cells. Also, bacteria can exchange genetic material with each other, fashioned into plasmids, the rings of DNA code. Normal human cells must make do with their original genes.

Humans contain some immortal cells—the germ cells that become egg, sperm and ultimately a new person. Germ cells differ from all other human cells because eggs and sperm have only half the normal complement of chromosomes. Of possibly even greater significance, germ cells divide in a special way—the process of meiosis described in an earlier chapter. Meiosis provides an opportunity to clean up any errors that might have gotten into the DNA. The genes contributed by two individuals almost always work better than the genes of any one person, no matter how fit or long-lived. This effect, called hybrid vigor, has frustrated most efforts to pinpoint longevity genes through inbreeding of longer-lived laboratory animals.

The life expectancy of laboratory animals bred for longevity can usually be increased by crossbreeding with *any* other strain. The reason probably has to do with the recessive genes described earlier. The inbred animals may acquire two copies of a longevity gene that is recessive and therefore doesn't have much effect unless two copies are present. But it also acquires duplicate copies of recessive genes that are harmful. As the animals are crossbred with another strain, all the recessive genes are diluted.

The powerful effect of combining the genes of two persons is another major reason that human germ cells are immortal and normal differentiated cells are not. Defective germ cells do occur, but the large majority are eliminated before conception or through spontaneous abortion. That leaves the human inheritance passed through the tough, immortal survivors of germ cells. The rest of us is constructed of less stern stuff and perishes in 115 years or less.

Cell biologists have searched hard to find the specific machinery in a normal human cell that might be responsible for the limit on 50 population doublings. Research has provided no firm answers, but it does reveal intriguing and provocative clues.

The other apparently immortal cells are cancer cells. A legendary strain of cervical cancer cells, code-named HeLa, has been alive since 1952 and has undergone many, many more population doublings than normal human cells. One of the tricks that cell biologists use to understand operations at the cellular level is to fuse two different cells together and observe what happens. In one experiment, normal but mortal human cells were fused with immortal cancer cells. As it turned out, the fused, combined cells were mortal, just like the normal human cells. Almost certainly this means that a gene in the normal cells is enforcing the limit, and this gene is a dominant gene—a single copy is enough. If normal young human fibroblasts are fused with old fibroblasts, the older cell's limit on cell division also prevails. The search for the location of these genes has been refined somewhat by fusing immortal cancer cells with altered cells that contain only a single human chromosome. Fusing a cell containing human chromosome 4 with an immortal cell is sufficient to return the cell line to mortal cell division limits. Injecting minute amounts of the cell fluid taken from old fibroblasts into immortal cancer cells also brings cell division to a halt. That suggests that one longevity-limiting gene contains the instructions for manufacturing a protein that, in very small quantities, halts cell division.

This line of inquiry might reveal either what happens to normal human cells to make them cancerous, or why cancerous cells are immortal. However, this doesn't necessarily mean that an elixir of eternal life beckons on the near research horizon. It could be, for example, that the limit on cell division provides a net benefit, and that's why it occurs. It's also possible that the limit on proliferation is part of a tradeoff for some other essential cell function. All this suggests that we're starting to take apart the engine of longevity for the first time. While each component part performs fascinating functions, that is hardly a guarantee we'll be able to build a better machine than the existing one, which has been perfected through billions of years of random experimentation.

Still, it is of great interest to examine what the component pieces of this engine might look like. Cell biologists are intensely curious about how human cells are able to count to 50 and know when to cease cell division. The mystery is deepened because apparently the cells of shorter-lived mammals undergo fewer cell divisions. Fibroblasts from a mouse embryo, for example, appear to double in culture from 14 to 28 times instead of 50 times. If this is confirmed, it makes it quite likely that the demise of cell proliferation is genetically programmed, and not the result of environmental damage. This is because mouse and human fibroblast cells, growing under identical circumstances in laboratory bottles, ought to suffer damage at the same rate.

The cells may in fact contain "a genetic time bomb," according to a theory advanced by Calvin B. Harley, a Canadian biochemist. He has an ingenious explanation of how cells keep count of divisions so as to recognize the end of useful life. The ends of individual chromosomes contain a sequence of repeating code, almost like a filler inserted after the last gene. These ends are called telomeres, and the same repeated sequence—abbreviated TTAGGG—is shared by creatures ranging from humans to slime mold. In this theory, each time a normal cell divides, about six letters of the telomere filler are lost when the DNA replicates. The enzyme that helps replicate cell DNA can't get the ends exactly right, and a little data is lost each time. Having an expendable filler sequence at the end is a workable solution, but after a certain number of cell divisions, the telomere will be gone, and operating genes might be damaged. It is also possible that as the chromosomes are accidentally shortened, the rough ends get sticky, and may accidentally fuse with another chromosome, creating an abnormal cell. Such chromosome abnormalities are found, for example, in Down's syndrome.

One intriguing fact supports Harley's theory. Immortal human germ cells—which produce the egg and the sperm—have apparently escaped this limitation, and are equipped with a special enzyme, telomerase, which permits DNA replication without snipping off the chromosome ends. Harley has also found that in old human fibroblasts, the telomeres are shorter. But the telomere remains only a tantalizing lead. Does this play a central causal role in aging, or is it simply another entry in the catalog of 200 known changes that occur in cell aging, some of which are significant, some of which are not?

Harley's is not the only theory swirling through the world of longevity research at the cellular level. Other researchers have isolated a family of growth inhibitors found in old fibroblasts that shut down cell division when injected into young fibroblasts. Another approach suggests that the loss of ability to divide is simply one result of a general decline in a cell's ability to manufacture a wide variety of different proteins.

An important but contrasting view emphasizes that immortal cells are abnormal cells, mainly cancer cells. To remain healthy, the body is equipped with a series of controls to limit cell division under most circumstances. The goal, therefore, is better enforcement of limits on cell division rather than tinkering with those limits. One important marker of the aging process is the abnormal proliferation of cells. Many of these abnormal cell proliferations are not cancerous—for example, the benign growth in the prostate of a majority of older men, formation of polyps in the intestine, or increased hair growth in the nose or ears that occurs with age.

In one important theory, abnormal cell growth is the seminal event in coronary heart disease as well as in cancer. The first step in the formation of the obstructions in the coronary arteries may occur when the smooth inner lining is damaged. The smooth muscle cells that line the arteries proliferate and intrude through the damaged lining to help form what later becomes a permanent and slowly expanding lesion. Those who have the most serious, and therefore life-threatening, obstructions are those with unusually large amounts of smooth muscle cell proliferation. Thus in this theory, the finite limits on cell division are part of the body's defenses against heart disease and cancer.

Man, however, does not live longer by theory alone. The next chapter will explore approaches to combating the aging process that have produced results in animals, or are being actually tested in humans. The world where real interventions are tested in complete organisms is much less tidy than the arena where ingenious theories are formulated and tested in model systems. But it may be no less likely to produce usable results, and some would argue more so.

CHAPTER FOURTEEN

PRACTICAL LONGEVITY

EXPERIMENTS

At a National Institutes of Health laboratory in Poolesville, Maryland, researchers are attempting to extend the maximum lifespan of two close human relatives, the rhesus and squirrel monkeys. It is a serious, carefully controlled test of an intervention intended to extend the reproductive period, the average lifespan and the maximum length of life. On repeated occasions, this technique has extended the maximum lifespan of rats and mice by 50 percent. One researcher who has experimented extensively with this technique, pathologist Roy L. Walford of the University of California at Los Angeles, has chosen to test it on himself. He has decided not to wait for the results of the Poolesville experiment, the first with animals more closely related to humans. The intervention is called diet restriction, and it requires a lifetime of going hungry.

Diet restriction, however, may reveal more about the current state of progress in the science of longevity than it does about the underlying nature of the aging process. Laboratory mice whose food intake is reduced by 25 to 60 percent will live longer than matched controls allowed to eat at will. This finding has been confirmed hundreds of times since the effects were first reported in 1934. However, in six decades of additional research, no comparable method of altering the mammalian lifespan has yet been discovered. Nor is it clear how diet restriction achieves its salutory effects.

This situation is reminiscent of Edward Jenner's discovery of smallpox vaccination in 1799. It was stunningly effective, but ignorance of the bedrock fundamentals of infectious disease meant no other vaccines were discovered for many decades—not until Louis Pasteur deduced the existence and functions of immunity, the fruit of many years of meticulous experiment and careful observation. Jenner discovered an isolated technique that ultimately led Pasteur to an idea of great power.

Diet restriction remains a technique. Nevertheless, it fuels the fires of possibility for those who would pursue a new power over the forces of life, those that control its length. Therefore, diet restriction, and the other practical interventions that will be explored in this chapter, suggest these fundamental and important characteristics of longevity research: It looks possible to extend the human lifespan, perhaps by decades. Unfortunately, this may not be easy, and will require the usual combination of brilliance, luck and tedious, systematic experimentation.

The technique of diet restriction is simple, but baffling; it is effective by numerous measures, but still mysterious after hundreds of attempts to unlock its inner secrets. A research team at the University of California at Los Angeles performed one of the classic demonstrations in 1986. The experiment was led by Richard Weindruch, who is now at the National Institute on Aging's research center in Baltimore. The subjects were 349 hybrid laboratory mice, the genetically similar—but not identical—offspring of two strains inbred for long-lived characteristics. The experiment began immediately after weaning at about three weeks of age. The mice lived their lives on a bed of wood chips in plastic cages housed in a room with unvarying temperature and humidity, and consistent hours of light and darkness. The 49 mice in the control group were free to consume unlimited amounts of Ralston Purina Laboratory Chow. The test animals were fed reduced amounts of a special diet of sugar, corn oil, fiber, and various vitamins and minerals. The most severely restricted group would get only 40 percent of the caloric intake of the control animals. The human equivalent would mean spending childhood, adolescence and adult life on a diet of 800 to 900 calories a day. The other mice got 50 to 75 percent of the control group's calories. No particular component of the special diet was believed to have life-prolonging properties. It was designed to provide all the essential proteins, minerals, carbohydrates and fat needed for life, but with greatly reduced total calories. In short, in this experiment a longevity diet was simply a well-balanced one featuring fewer calories. In fact, the same effect has been observed where the diet-restricted group was fed standard laboratory chow on alternate days.

The first mouse to die was in the control group that ate what it wanted, succumbing at just 6 months of age. But this was merely an example of a premature death that occurs in all animal populations, and probably had nothing to do with the aging process itself. Under these controlled conditions such deaths were rare: just 4 in the first 20 months of life. Then relentless exponential growth of mortality rates began to tell, and by 36 months there were no survivors. However, at this point when not one member of the control group survived, all but 4 of the 60 mice on the most severely restricted diet were still alive. The longest-lived diet-restricted mouse survived 55 months—an increase in maximum lifespan of 55 percent. The life expectancy, or average length of life, showed similar improvement. On the average, the control group lived 27 months; the diet-restriction group 45 months. This is a significant shift of the entire mortality curve under well-controlled conditions. The results of different degrees of calorie restriction vary in tidy fashion according to the severity of the diet; the fewer the calories the better, but only to a certain point. The experimenters believed that any more severe diet restriction might have quickly killed the animals.

Simply demonstrating the effect of diet restriction does not answer a pivotal question: Is the aging process itself being retarded? Some theorists—for example, the National Institute on Aging's Barry Cutler—argue such experiments do not prove the lifespan of a mammal has been increased. The truly normal mice, he noted, are those on diet restriction, getting limited quantities of food much as they would get in the wild. The abnormal animals are those confined in small cages and offered unlimited amounts of food.

Without a uniform measure of aging—and reliable indicators to mark its progress—Cutler's objection cannot be set aside. However, reasonably convincing evidence exists suggesting that the aging process itself appears to be affected in this experiment. Evidence does not depend solely on the fact that diet-restricted animals typically live longer. Chronic life-terminating disorders such as kidney failure and cancer are also postponed. The animals have an extended reproductive life. Deterioration of memory with age is deferred. Hormone levels of old restricted mice resemble those of younger mice fed on demand. Mice that are deliberately inbred for vulnerability to disorders such as mammary or lymphatic cancer develop these diseases at later ages. Deterioration of the immune system is postponed. If these are really just experiments that prove overfeeding is harmful to caged mice, then excess food certainly causes an enormous array of ill effects.

The demonstration of an effect on longevity would be more convincing and immensely more valuable if accompanied by a clear explanation for how these effects are achieved. That question has not yet been answered. Literally decades of research have been more successful in eliminating theories than in confirming one of them. The specific foods used in the various experiments have varied so widely that either harmful or beneficial effects of a particular nutrient have been ruled out.

For many years researchers believed the main effects of diet restriction were in delaying the arrival of sexual maturity—in short, slowing only the development phase of life cycle. But recent experiments have proved that diet restriction imposed on mature adults also extends the lifespan—although the earlier the diet begins, the greater the impact.

Others believed the benefits came because the very lean diet completely eliminated any ill effects of obesity. This explanation was laid to rest in an experiment that included some animals with such a strong genetic predisposition to obesity that they got fat even on a restricted diet. This experiment showed that the amount of body fat didn't have any effect on lifespan—the factor that mattered was food intake.

Finally many researchers thought that fewer calories of food simply slowed down the body metabolism. This underlying theory suggests that the cells can complete only a fixed number of chemical reactions before damage and deterioration occur. The less energy available from food, the slower the metabolism and the longer the cells survive. But in a key experiment, Edward J. Masoro of the University of Texas showed that metabolism apparently wasn't slowed in diet-restricted animals, even though less total energy was available from food. The restricted animals utilized calories more efficiently—and reduced their body mass so as to require fewer of them.

The surviving theories suggest the longevity benefit may lie in the hormonal response to the signals of starvation. It is possible that cell functions throughout the body are changed by the hormonal chemical messengers secreted in response to starvation. Which hormones are the important ones—and how they achieve a life-prolonging effect—remains to be determined. If confirmed, hormonal theories might open

the door to human interventions that don't require a lifetime of exposure to the body's starvation alarms. Hormones could be synthesized and
provided in daily doses, just as thyroid and female sex hormones are
routinely prescribed today.

Would a lifetime of diet restriction lengthen the human lifespan? The
evidence in human adults is mixed. By some measures, prolonged dieting in adults produces an array of apparently beneficial health effects.
Reducing calorie intake lowers blood pressure, serum cholesterol and
blood sugar levels. But as was seen in earlier chapters on the risk factor
diseases, the effects tend to be small. In a 1992 study of blood pressure
reduction without drugs, a diet severe enough to sustain 9-pound
weight losses for six months reduced blood pressure only by 2.7 percent.
As noted earlier, blood pressure reductions of roughly double this magnitude achieved with drugs reduced the incidence of strokes but had
little or no effect on coronary heart disease and total mortality. Choles-
terol-reducing diets with 15 to 21 percent reduction in calories typically
reduced cholesterol levels by 2 to 7 percent, but achieved no change in
premature mortality. Dieting reduces blood sugar in those with elevated
levels, but the overall effect on mortality status is unknown. The two
World Wars effectively imposed diet restriction on the populations of
entire European countries. In World War II, mortality rates fell among
noncombatants in several countries, notably England and Denmark. But
in World War I, reduced amounts of meat and dairy products were
blamed for raising mortality rates—especially from tuberculosis and
other infectious diseases.

Meanwhile, the initial results are promising but certainly not conclusive in the diet-restriction experiments among 93 rhesus and squirrel
monkeys that are caged in Poolesville, Maryland. The monkeys could
not tolerate as severe a restriction as laboratory rats, says George Roth,
who directs the experiments for the National Institute on Aging. The
restricted monkeys receive 25 percent fewer calories, which is near the
minimum cutback needed to achieve an effect in rodents. However, the
restricted young animals gained weight more slowly, and the restricted
juveniles reached puberty about one year later than those with unlimited
food available. While hundreds of thousands of dollars are being spent
in hopes that diet restriction will work in primates, Roth warns that
success is by no means guaranteed. "It could be that the response was an

evolutionary adaptation in rodents that allowed them to survive an extra year when food might be more plentiful. This might be irrelevant in long-lived mammals." Another possible outcome is that the effect will occur in primates but add the same number of months to lifespan as in mice. Ten months amounts to a 50 percent increase for a mouse, but would be too small to detect in an experiment with fewer than 100 monkeys.

However, one possible effect of diet is now being tested in tens of thousands of humans. Diet is one of several factors that may also retard one of the most fundamental of all chemical processes—oxidation.

If the validity of longevity theories were measured by the number of people willing to test an intervention on themselves, then it must be concluded that antioxidants play a pivotal role in the aging process. Millions of people take special preparations of vitamin C, vitamin E, selenium or beta-carotene; many millions more have altered their diet to eat more fruits and vegetables that are naturally rich in these chemicals. One mechanism through which antioxidants might prolong life is by reducing the incidence of cancer. This possibility is taken so seriously that the National Cancer Institute is now sponsoring seven controlled clinical trials with tens of thousands of carefully monitored participants. A book touting the virtues of antioxidants, *Life Extension,* was a million-copy best seller.

While the use of antioxidants constitutes one of the most popular of all interventions for increasing life expectancy, its critics believe it involves such a fundamental problem of biochemistry that all viable life-forms solved it hundreds of millions of years ago. It all has to do with containing the potentially lethal effects of one of the wellsprings of life, oxygen.

The use of antioxidants stems from the free radical theory of aging, whose roots lie in basic chemistry. Free radicals might be described as molecular mischief-makers. Their outer shells are missing one or two electrons, giving them a strong affinity for the whirling electrons of other, more stable molecules. As a consequence, free radicals engage in a chemical reaction that transforms both the free radical and the otherwise stable molecule. This might alter a molecule in a cell that was needed to perform some useful function. The essential and ubiquitous element oxygen happens to have exactly the right nuclear configuration to form free radicals. As a plentiful atmospheric gas, O_2, it has two unpaired electrons and tries to pair with surrounding molecules, a process called oxidation. The most dramatic exhibition of rapid oxidation is called fire. A slower and more gradual version of the process is rust. These examples help illustrate that oxygen is potentially toxic because of its chemical capacity to transform either a block of unpainted iron or a fragile cell membrane. In the 1940s, physicians were puzzled by the damaged eyes found in many premature babies. The eye lenses, they discovered, were being oxidized by excessive concentrations of oxygen provided in the incubators.

The chemical properties of free radicals fascinated a young American chemistry student named Denham Harmon. He became so fascinated by the role they might play in living systems that he went to medical school specifically to pursue this interest. Then, in 1954, he proposed that unwanted chemical reactions triggered by free radicals lay at the heart of the process of aging. It was a bold, intriguing and mostly unprovable theory that attracted a small band of loyal followers, but otherwise was mostly disregarded. The problem was that most free radical molecules existed only for a tiny fraction of a second before being transformed into a more stable structure. So they could not be readily observed, measured or detected in living cells. Nevertheless, evidence slowly accumulated that free radicals could, at least in theory, wreak havoc inside a cell. They could scramble the genetic code in DNA. They seemed capable of wrecking the finely balanced gatekeeping functions of cell membranes. They might disrupt the mitochondria, the tiny units within a cell that supply energy. Basic chemistry suggested these things could happen. But did they?

William A. Pryor, a biochemist at Louisiana State University, has developed a model system that illustrates the mischief-making capacity of oxygen-based free radicals. A single free radical triggers a kind of domino effect when set loose among molecules of an essential fat compound, linoleic acid. A single free radical, Pryor calculated, would wreck about 26 molecules of linoleic acid before the reaction stopped. But free radicals can be created by many natural events—by sunlight, by radiation, and as a by-product of internal chemical reactions triggered by cell enzymes. Free radicals would quickly destroy the cells without a defense, but it turns out that cell defenses can be dramatically effective. When the linoleic acid was mixed with vitamin E in Pryor's experiment, the chain reaction quickly sputtered out—the biological equivalent of a bucket of water thrown on a bed of smoldering coals.

Cells are loaded with antioxidants, for example, vitamin E, vitamin C, vitamin A, beta-carotene and glutathione peroxidase. Some metals, notably selenium, also have antioxidant properties, and other metals, for example, iron, facilitate chemical reactions that help form damaging free radicals. The discovery of so many cellular antioxidants fueled the arguments of both proponents and critics of the free radical theory. Adherents were delighted to discover hard evidence that the chemical reactions involving free radicals were indeed a central threat to cells. Why else would so many mechanisms exist to neutralize them? Skeptics said this was evidence the problem was solved two billion years ago, when the earliest plants flooded the atmosphere with increasing concentrations of oxygen created through photosynthesis. Proponents have suggested that free radicals may play a role in cancer, heart disease, aging, cataracts, emphysema, kidney disease, liver failure, dementia, arthritis and osteoporosis. Critics want to see the proof.

For almost forty years the free radical theory of aging has resembled an active ghost in the proverbial haunted house, leaving mysterious traces everywhere, but elusive and extremely difficult to pin down. In the 1960s, the father of the free radical theory, Denham Harmon, fed large amounts of antioxidants to laboratory rodents. Fewer premature deaths occurred, but the entire mortality curve was not shifted, as in diet restriction. Also, critics argued that damage from free radicals ought to occur at uniform rates throughout life, creating an entirely different pattern from the rapid upward sweep of mortality rates observed late in life.

Just as interest was dwindling in the free radical approach, the enzyme superoxide dismutase, or SOD, was discovered in 1969. Finding that cells manufacture an enzyme whose only purpose is to inhibit a specific form of free radical oxygen, called superoxide, gave the theory a whole new lease on life. It proved that free radicals were a serious enough peril to cell function that an antidote had to be kept immediately at hand. And older cells tended to have less superoxide dismutase. So perhaps aging was not a direct result of free radical damage, but of a decline of cellular defenses. In one of those blind leaps of faith that are often found on the fringes of longevity research, some people included SOD in their diet in hopes of bolstering declining supplies inside the cells. This was a pointless exercise, however, because superoxide dismutase is broken down during digestion.

Some diet enthusiasts also embraced foods loaded with the antioxidant mineral selenium. It is required for another free radical scavenging mechanism involving the enzyme glutathione peroxidase. Total absence of selenium from the diet has been implicated in extremely rare degenerative heart and bone disorders observed only in isolated areas of China and Korea. However, Western diets contain more than adequate amounts of selenium, according to Barry Halliwell, a British biochemist and authority on free radicals. And, he notes, larger amounts can be toxic, causing the hair and fingernails to fall out.

To survey the literature on free radicals is to discover a subject rich in possibilities and tantalizing clues, but without conclusive intervention studies in animals or humans. However, at least one property of antioxidants has looked promising enough to spur major trials involving thousands of human subjects. Taking antioxidants just might help prevent cancer. At least as measured by the thousands of individuals taking it in controlled trials, beta-carotene is the leading candidate for an antioxidant that works. Beta-carotene is found in plants and vegetables; in the human body it is converted into vitamin A. Studies of lung cancer victims suggested that not only did they tend to be heavy smokers, but they had lower-than-average levels of beta-carotene in their blood. In theory, at least, this is a potentially lethal combination, because cigarette smoke is rich in long-lived free radicals, and vitamin A is one of the free radical scavengers. The National Cancer Institute is currently sponsoring ten clinical trials to see whether beta-carotene might help prevent several forms of cancer, particularly lung cancer. Two of the experiments focus on individuals at very high risk for lung cancer—heavy smokers and heavy smokers who were also exposed to asbestos.

The largest and oldest controlled experiment involved 22,000 physicians, serving as test subjects to measure the effect of taking two different pills, aspirin and beta-carotene, on alternate days. But one of the two pills each physician took was in fact a placebo, allowing researchers to measure separately the effect of each. The aspirin component of the trial attracted worldwide attention in 1987 when researchers reported those taking the aspirin had 40 percent fewer heart attacks than those getting the placebo. (However, there was no difference in overall deaths between the doctors taking aspirin or taking the placebo. Either the effect on life expectancy was too small to be measured in this large study, or taking the aspirin reduced the risk of heart attack but increased the risk of other disorders.) Although the effects on heart attacks were widely publicized, hardly anyone noticed that beta-carotene had no measurable effect at the end of five years. The trial was therefore extended an additional five years. No measurable effects were obtained at the 10-year mark in 1990, and the trial was extended for still another five years in hopes of achieving a successful result—or perhaps to postpone admitting that the experiment had failed. Winfred F. Malone, the chief of the Chemoprevention Branch of the National Cancer Institute, conceded that if beta-carotene ultimately produces a preventive role in cancer, it is likely to be a small effect, perhaps a 10 percent reduction in risk. The effects, however, might be more important in high-risk individuals, such as smokers, or in those who take a combination of beta-carotene and other antioxidants. But as this is written there is no evidence of efficacy from human intervention trials, and a mixture of failure and success in animal experiments.

After nearly four decades of research, compelling evidence has accumulated that free radicals are capable of causing harm to biological systems, corrupting DNA, damaging cell membranes and short-circuiting the cell's energy cycle. But that same research has increasingly revealed the sophisticated nature of cell defenses. It is possible that free radicals are cancer promoters, nurturing the mutated cells that are just beginning to escape the body's control. It is also conceivable that free radicals play a key role in coronary heart disease as the mechanism through which the smooth inner surfaces of arteries are first damaged. What makes the free radical theory so hard to confirm or disprove is the many different roles that these molecules *might* play. This is a prime example of what makes longevity science a world of paradox, featuring so many intriguing clues but so little hard evidence.

At the opposite end of the intellectual spectrum from the sprawling and unruly free radical theory is an inexpensive chemical of known structure that seems to have a dazzling array of nearly miraculous properties.

At first glance, the claims for this possible wonder drug would look more at home in a supermarket tabloid than in publications such as *Brain Research* or the *Journal of Clinical Endocrinology and Metabolism*. Not even jargon-loving professionals try to pronounce the name of this substance—dehydroepiandosterone. It is called DHEA for short and is a human steroid hormone first isolated in 1934. The natural function and purpose of DHEA, the most plentiful hormone in the human body, remain unknown to this day. However, it has one characteristic that immediately captures the interest of longevity researchers. DHEA levels in the bloodstream reach a maximum at age 25, and then decline steadily throughout the rest of life. It could be simply a coincidence. But here is the mirror image of the central force of mortality, which begins its exponential rise just as DHEA levels decline.

In animal studies, DHEA appears to reverse numerous effects associated with aging. For example, it has antiobesity properties in laboratory mice genetically predisposed to gain weight. Mice given DHEA got leaner without reducing their food intake. In laboratory cultures, DHEA protects rat and hamster cells from chemically induced cancer. In living mice, DHEA has been shown to inhibit spontaneous breast cancer, as well as thyroid, skin, liver and colon tumors intentionally induced by chemicals. The breast cancer finding was of particular interest because some studies suggest that DHEA levels are depressed among women with breast cancer. A single study in laboratory mice suggests DHEA might slow the process underlying coronary heart disease. A lone epidemiological study reported elevated risks of coronary heart disease among humans with lower-than-average levels of DHEA. The hormone enhanced memory retention in mice, reversing the effects of amnesia deliberately induced with chemicals. Also in laboratory mice, DHEA appears to strengthen the immune system response to viruses. In the single experiment in the literature, mice were injected with one of two potentially lethal viruses, producing 88 to 90 percent mortality in untreated animals. In comparable groups of animals injected with DHEA, all survived infections from one virus, and 63 percent survived the other. Finally, DHEA produced rapid remission of diabetes in mice genetically predisposed to the disorder.

Can this be? A human hormone that might inhibit cancer, heart disease and diabetes while enhancing both memory retention and the immune response to viral infections? DHEA, however, is not without some known limitations. As its name suggests, it is a steroid hormone secreted by the adrenal glands, and it happens to be a precursor of testosterone, the male sex hormone. DHEA, therefore, may be converted into sex hormones in the body and may thereby lose some of its effectiveness. In immature mice it caused atrophy of the uterus in females and enlargement of the sperm-holding vesicles in males. However, a synthetic variant of DHEA has been developed that cannot be converted to sex hormones, and it is apparently more effective in nonsexual properties. Animal models using mice inbred for vulnerability to breast cancer, diabetes or other disorders are an excellent way to test for effects of large doses of a chemical. Such experiments, however, are only the beginning of a long journey toward demonstrating a useful effect of DHEA in humans.

It is nevertheless surprising how slowly knowledge of DHEA has developed since its beneficial properties were first publicized more than a decade ago. There have been no large-scale experiments in humans and only a few continuing studies in animals. In a world where biological research is booming, why has interest been so limited in DHEA?

Winfred Malone, who heads cancer prevention studies at the National Cancer Institute, said his office was funding a preliminary study to determine the effects of administering the new synthetic version of DHEA to a small number of people. The first step is to test its safety. So the National Cancer Institute remains interested, although this is a small-scale project.

Richard Sprott, the associate director who supervises the award of research grants for the National Institute on Aging, said that the institute gets very few applications for DHEA research. Sprott offered to hold a conference to assemble all the world's DHEA experts to compare results and stimulate new research. He made the offer almost ten years ago, he said, and it is still open.

The limited interest in DHEA is also mystifying to the man who developed the synthetic version of the hormone, Arthur G. Schwartz, of Temple Medical School in Philadelphia. "It's not in the mainstream," he said. "This is a steroid and this is simply not a hot area." He got also poor response when he tried to interest drug companies. "I was told flat out by a major drug company that they were not interested in cancer prevention," Schwartz said. "If they were, they would go with this drug." In Europe today, DHEA is sold over the counter. In the doses in which it is provided, Schwartz is doubtful that it would have a beneficial effect.

Meanwhile, Schwartz began testing his synthetic version in a few human subjects in the summer of 1992. But the biggest question about DHEA remains unanswered. "Nobody knows what the biological function of DHEA is," said Schwartz.

More is known about another hormone with apparent antiaging properties. When first tested in elderly men, it was credited with reversing some effects of 20 years of aging in just a few months. One of eight important hormones secreted by the pituitary gland, it is called human growth hormone. Low levels of growth hormone in children produces dwarfism, and the hormone has been given for many years to prevent this disorder. But growth hormone is secreted throughout life—in daily pulses occurring mostly at night. It stimulates the growth of many kinds of tissue, causes the reduction of body fat and increases the lean mass of muscle, bone and other organs. Growth hormone levels decline with age in some but not all adults. It is thought to be a factor in the decrease in muscle and lean body mass and the increase in fat that are observed with advancing age.

In an experiment that received national news media attention, Daniel Rudman, of the Medical College of Wisconsin, gave the hormone to 12 healthy elderly men with low natural levels of human growth hormone. The treatment—which costs roughly $13,000 a year and involves three injections per week—seemed to reverse the gradual atrophy of muscle, bone, liver and skin that occurs over 10 to 20 years. Here was a substance that, at first blush, appeared to reverse an important effect of aging when growth hormone levels were raised to the level of healthy young adults. Although the hormonally linked changes in fat distribution, muscle and bone were probably not some central mechanism of aging, many individuals might be eager to reverse these effects alone.

Since human growth hormone occurs naturally and has been given routinely to children, it offered a promising initial reputation for safety. However, little is known about the long-term effects of growth hormone replacement, nor have ideal levels been established. Excess secretions of growth hormone are a well-documented genetic disorder called acromegaly, and can cause gigantism, high blood pressure, accelerated coronary heart disease, diabetes and premature death.

Human growth hormone remains another of those promising leads in longevity research. It might prove to have great value in a wide range of individuals, and more thorough study might also reveal side effects that outweigh the benefits for most people. Or human growth hormone might ultimately be among those hormones replaced in only those individuals with deficiencies. This occurs routinely today with thyroid hormones. Since the central mechanism of aging remains mysterious, many would be content to counter the effects of aging, one by one. In their heart of hearts, humans have never accepted aging as inevitable, nor been satisfied with the lifespan that nature seems to provide. It is said to be a considerable achievement to age gracefully. Nevertheless, the search continues for the tools with which to slow down this process as much as possible.

CHAPTER FIFTEEN

A SUMMING UP

When it comes to the subject of longevity, some of the people are fooled all of the time, and we are all fools once in a while. Under the best of circumstances, it is hard to steer a steady course through this unusual subject, which combines such a strange mix of hopes, fact, fears and uncertainty. As earlier chapters illustrated, much of the information about longevity in daily circulation is provided by parties with another motive besides providing a balanced view about an inherently emotional subject. The cast with its own separate agenda includes zealous health activists, ambitious medical bureaucrats and profiteers relying on the cynical manipulation of the fear of dying. All this complicates the task of this final chapter—exploring how to balance the longevity choices in life.

This book was never intended to tell you what to do. If anything, it has been dedicated to demonstrating that too much health advice has been provided without an adequate scientific foundation. It would only compound the problem to provide an additional set of unsubstantiated judgments. And after all, it little behooves the author who cries, "The emperor has no clothes," to proceed immediately to don his jacket. There are, however, basic principles everyone can apply, and some obvious mistakes to avoid.

Because this book contains generous amounts of criticism of the national medical authorities and the public health community, it is likely to be criticized for doctor-bashing. It was intended as a partial remedy for a general failure to examine the strengths and weaknesses of the medical care system with the same wary caution with which, for example, the military-industrial complex has long been viewed. We know that the Defense Department is essential. But we also know it is prone to excess, to desire too many or too fancy weapons for the actual threat at hand. But the military is also peopled by dedicated individuals who perform bravely when we need them. This is no less true of the world of medicine, except our fears about longevity are so great that medical excesses are seldom brought into clear focus. A more balanced perspective on questions of longevity automatically encourages a more realistic view of the kinds of tasks the medical system performs spectacularly well and those it does poorly. In short, we are all more likely to be reasonable about doctors if we are not being fools about longevity.

A single, sobering analogy outlines the fundamentals of the great game of longevity. It has just two basic features, a longevity account and a lottery. Suppose everyone had a special account, with regular withdrawals and contributions made in accordance with the achievements and vicissitudes of life—something like a personal version of a stock mutual fund. However, no one starts life with exactly the same account balance. Throughout life everyone makes a series of deposits and withdrawals, and everyone has different results with the funds accumulated. This is the easy part, and it conforms to our intuitive sense of how life works.

Now comes the uncomfortable part of the longevity game. Every year a lottery is held under such favorable odds that the overwhelming majority always emerge as winners. But the losers die. At any particular age, the overall results of the lottery are known with great precision. For example out of 2,000 women in this lottery at age 20, just one will die, leaving 1,999 winners. By age 50, the lottery still returns 1,992 winners. A total of 1,934 of those who play at age 75 will win. And out of 2,000 who reach age 90, there will be 1,709 winners. As can be observed, even at a very advanced age, most people still win the longevity lottery. But at the heart of the oldest dream lies the human desire not to be forced to play this game at all. Unfortunately many people spend a good portion of their lives either foolishly pretending that these risks do not exist, or paralyzed with anxiety over the inescapable requirement to play. It is more productive to face reality knowing that for most of us, most of the time, the odds are pretty good.

The figures above are the overall odds for the game of life, as tabulated for all women in the United States in 1988. However, the chances for every individual will be different, and depend on the exact balance in the longevity account. However, as far as anyone can tell, no one has figured out any workable method of making contributions to one's own longevity fund large enough to overcome the steadily increasing account withdrawals mandated by advancing age. But individual choices and actions do indeed make a difference.

Consider the effect of the best documented and most easily avoidable major hazard of everyday life, smoking cigarettes. A heavy smoking habit is the equivalent of reducing your longevity account balance every year by an extra 12 percent. The odds in the lottery are good enough that most smokers still emerge as winners. But if we start counting about age 25, heavy smokers will lose an annual lottery an average of seven years earlier than those who never smoked. Some of those who don't smoke will still die at an early age, and some smokers will pass age 90.

We also know that women either are endowed with larger account balances or make slower annual withdrawals, putting them about 15 percent ahead of men. In the United States, the circumstances of life levy much larger annual withdrawals from the accounts of blacks compared with whites. Once again, a large annual difference of about 15 percent. The fundamental properties of longevity, therefore, are observed in the interplay of uncontrollable events and the consequences of individual human action. Most people are far more comfortable facing the consequences of their own actions than living with the certain prospect that their best efforts are subject to a throw of the dice.

Cigarette smoking is one of the few cases where the contributions and withdrawals from the longevity account can be calculated with some precision. Most of the other interventions described in this book involve mixtures of harm and benefit that differ among individuals. Often the net effect is extremely hard to determine, or has never been calculated. Most people seem to have an intuitive sense of the balance in their own longevity account, especially as it starts to get small. But it has thus far proved impossible to measure this scientifically and objectively.

The search for biomarkers of aging is one form of this effort. We are mostly confined to epidemiological studies that count the winners and losers of the lottery and try to infer, secondhand, what the account balances might have been. Then researchers try to measure the effects of an intervention, again trying to measure accurately despite the random interference introduced by the intervening lottery. As the numerous studies reported earlier demonstrate, it requires observing thousands of individuals for many years to record even a modest measurable effect. Partly this is because the chances of losing the lottery are so small that large numbers are required to observe a representative group of unfortunate losers. Partly it is because the effects of the interventions in question were in fact quite small. Everyone would love a panacea with dramatic effects. In truth, most contributions and withdrawals from the longevity account occur unceasingly, but in quite small amounts.

Most of us, therefore, would be better off cultivating and trusting our instincts. Some people might be healthier and happier if they stopped a hated jogging regimen and spent the time with a community or church group; for someone near victory in a battle with excess weight, exercise might be the key to success. Some people ought to spend more time with their family; others desperately need time for themselves. There are individuals who glory in risk taking, and those who need to play it safe. We all know of people who by grace of good fortune were born with a lot of longevity advantages, and by dint of hard work enhanced them. Others learned early the hard way that life is not fair, and that they must labor unrelentingly to compensate for biological, social or economic disadvantages. Given balanced information about hazards to health, most people will make reasonable choices for themselves. They probably won't be perfect choices, and a few people will make terrible mistakes. But it is like freedom of speech. So great are its benefits that we readily accept that such freedom also allows statements that are false, foolish, stupid or destructive.

Although some heavily promoted interventions turn out to have a notably smaller effect than advertised, this does not mean that nothing matters, or that individual actions are inconsequential. Life probably offers many, many more actions with a beneficial effect on longevity than the handful being currently promoted. However, it appears the effect of each is quite modest. And most individuals would be happier and healthier choosing a way of life to suit themselves rather than slavishly trying to follow simplistic prescriptions being promoted by organizations with other agendas.

The final dimension of longevity involves not what we do as individuals, but the joint efforts of families, communities and nations over many years' time. It is the achievements of stable, prosperous democracies, over many decades of continuing effort, that have produced the best odds in human history for all their unwilling lottery players. And the single greatest long-term hazard to longevity—a breakdown in our now mostly harmonious relationship with microscopic forms of life—can only be managed, or mismanaged, on the level of community, nation and world. Societies are far more durable than any individuals, and survive periods where withdrawals exceed contributions. But as the republics of the former Soviet Union have illustrated, empires do indeed collapse from neglect, drastically reducing the opportunities for all the players involved. One cannot observe events in the United States without wondering about the ultimate consequences of the increasing pursuit of personal advantage at any cost while mortgaging our future as a nation and community. Many individuals believe their influence on public events is so small that they can ignore their responsibility to contribute to the larger common good. This attitude is no more useful or realistic than trying to pretend there is no lottery. It just increases the number of losers.

If the study of longevity reveals any central and enduring lesson, it is that securing a longer and healthier life is not something that will be achieved primarily by individual actions—be they hormone injections, jogging or megavitamins. By its very nature, longevity is something that we can achieve together, not only for ourselves, but for our children and our neighbors.

ACKNOWLEDGMENTS

To try to put into perspective a subject as vast as human longevity is a continuing lesson in how much even the simplest conclusions depend on the thoughts, ideas and work of hundreds of others. The contributions of the following individuals were of special note and great value:

BOOK ONE: LONGEVITY GAINS. Emily W. Carrow, Ph.D., until recently a virologist for the Food and Drug Administration, was kind enough to review the entire section. James Cawley, MPH, PAC, shared his ideas and his course materials on infectious disease for the M.P.H. program at George Washington University. James A. Curtin, M.D., the chief of medicine at Washington Hospital Center, generously allowed me to observe infection control in the hospital setting, and provided invaluable insights.

BOOK TWO: RISE OF THE RISK FACTOR DISEASES. John H. Laragh, M.D., Cornell University Medical College, provided invaluable guidance on hypertension and reviewed an earlier version of that chapter. C. Wayne Callaway, M.D., Ph.D., a Washington endocrine and metabolic disorder specialist, helped me understand obesity; and Michael Oliver, M.D., Britain's premier cholesterol researcher, provided many key insights into that subject.

BOOK THREE: THE SCIENCE OF LONGEVITY. Many of the perspectives on the aging process at the cellular level came from George R. Martin, Ph.D., director of the National Institute on Aging's Gerontology Research Center. He proved an invaluable guide through the complex literature on this subject.

The public-spirited insurance actuary Edward Lew generously shared his insights and copies of his studies; his many publications were an important source for this book.

As might be expected, those named above did not necessarily interpret the evidence on this vast and controversial subject the same way I did. Nevertheless, their critiques and suggestions were invaluable.

For a second time, George Washington University has provided a stimulating and hospitable environment in which to write a book. For this opportunity I'm particularly indebted to Roderick S. French, Ph.D., vice president for academic affairs, and Peter Budetti, M.D., J.D., director of the Center for Health Policy Research. The most heavily used university resource was the Himmelfarb medical library, where George Paul provided invaluable assistance in locating so many of the publications.

Finally, this book could not have been written without the effective efforts of my agent, Esther Newberg, and the interest and support of my editor at Simon & Schuster, Bob Bender.

Information about longevity unfortunately is not contained in a tidy collection of easily accessed publications. Instead it is spread throughout several scientific disciplines, including history, demography, biology, epidemiology, actuarial science and medicine. To assist others who want to explore this issue on their own, this notes section includes not only scholarly documentation but also other sources not specifically cited in the text.

Three authors had great influence in shaping this entire work. The biggest intellectual debt is owed to the great René Dubos, especially his landmark book, *The Mirage of Health*. Those interested in mortality risks for practically every known condition should consult Edward Lew's massive two-volume work, *Medical Risks*. It is a good starting point for locating the literature on hundreds of different specialized subjects. A provocative and intellectually satisfying examination of the issues involving the biology of aging can be found in Alex Comfort's *The Biology of Senescence*. Unfortunately, Dubos's book is almost forty years old and Comfort's is approaching fifteen.

Since this book also contains a separate bibliography for book-length materials, these sources will be cited in abbreviated academic style with author's last name and year, for example: Comfort (1979). Government publications without a meaningful named author will be indicated by short title. Scientific journals are cited by first author, journal, year, volume and starting page, for example: R. Reiser, *American Journal of Clinical Nutrition* (1984), 40:654. To facilitate electronic data searches, special care was used to include first name and middle initial exactly as shown in the publication. Two journals are abbreviated, the *Journal of the American Medical Association,* as *JAMA,* and the *New England Journal of Medicine,* as *NEJM.*

1. DIMENSIONS OF THE OLDEST DREAM

The average lifespan of 15–17 years for prehistoric man is based on the earliest known group of skeletons from neolithic times. Exceptionally high infant mortality brings down the average to make it seem like this population didn't live long enough to reproduce, which of course it did. See Chapter 3 for a more detailed discussion.

Examples of one night's advertising fare on the evening news included margarine, breakfast cereal, aspirin, antacids, and laxatives. Promotions concerning cholesterol and high blood pressure will be explained in the chapters on those subjects.

The mortality rate comparisons were taken primarily from John E. Sutherland, *JAMA* (1990), 264:3178. Also see the appropriate volumes of *Vital Statistics of the United States.* Changes in the definitions of diseases, notably coronary heart disease, introduce imperfections into any mortality comparisons prior to the current revision of the International Classification of Disease codes enacted in 1979. The main effect was a one-time increase in the reported incidence of coronary heart disease. The mortality figures for 10-year-old children came from the life table in *Statistical Abstracts of the United States,* 1991, Table 107. For 10-year-old white females, the rate is almost down to 1 in 10,000. The life expectancy of men and women nonsmokers in good health was adapted from Edward Lew's smoking study described below, but adjusted to current life expectancy. Dr. Richard Riegelman's story was told to me in a personal conversation. The fundamentals of the life table and other calculations can be found in Trowbridge (1989). A simple exposition of life table math appears in Chapter 3 of Arking (1991). The authoritative guide to mortality (versus life table) mathematics is found in the 1900–1940 volume of *Vital Statistics of the United States,* beginning at Chapter 4. The calculations for the table showing the time until 1 percent died were made by the author from the 1987 life table for the United States using the stationary population column. The chances of early teenagers dying came from 1987, *Vital Statistics of the United States.*

Edward Lew wrote many articles based on his landmark study of one million Americans, which he performed for the American Cancer Society. The summary quoted here came from Lew, *Transactions, Society of Actuaries* (1987), 39:107. The figures for women dying prematurely came from Richard G. Rogers, *Social Science Medicine* (1991), 32:1151. The twins study was from D. Carmelli, *Psychosomatic Medicine* (1988), 50:165. The smoking literature is summarized at enormous length in a series of reports from the United States Surgeon General, which are issued annually in thick volumes. The 1989 volume, *Reducing the Health Consequences of Smoking*, has a valuable historical section. The original analysis that launched the war against smoking was published in 1964 as *Smoking and Health: Report of the Advisory Committee to the Surgeon General of the Public Health Service*.

The international comparisons between the sexes came from the *U.S. Census World Population Profile*, 1989. A study of sex differences over the long term came in Barnet N. Berin, *Transactions, Society of Actuaries* (1989), 41:9. A thorough examination of biological advantages of modern women was written by Edward Dolnick. An excerpt appeared on page 11 in *The Washington Post*'s health weekly section, August 13, 1991.

The military mortality figures are from page 4–59 of Lew (1990). The Army is reported separately in Joseph M. Rothenberg, *JAMA* (1990), 264:2241. However, anyone who thinks military service is safe might review an analysis of mortality in war, Richard M. Garfield, *JAMA* (1991), 266:688. Mortality rates among the workers at Oak Ridge National Laboratory were reported in Steve Wing, *JAMA* (1991), 265:1397.

Ralph S. Paffenberger wrote several reports from his study of exercise habits of Harvard alumni. The figures in the chapter were in Ralph S. Paffenberger, *NEJM* (1986), 314:605. For cardiovascular risk see his study in *American Journal of Epidemiology* (1978), 108:161. Examples of Paffenberger's work being cited as an authority to promote exercise can be found in Jeffrey P. Koplan, JAMA (1989), 262:2437. The title, "Physical Activity, Physical Fitness, and Health: Time to Act," says it all. Also see a special section, "Public Health Aspects of Physical Activity and Exercise," in *Public Health Reports* (1985), 100:118. Arking (1991) reviews exercise to reverse muscular atrophy on page 267. For the increasing number of the individuals physically unable to exercise at older ages see the U.S. Center for Health Statistics' Health Interview Survey, which is reported annually.

The international life expectancy and fertility figures were quoted from the Census Bureau's *World Population Profile, 1989.* It differs slightly from the other major reference, the World Health Organization's *1989 World Health Statistics Annual,* and several countries share third place with Greece. The food consumption data came from the United Nations Food and Agriculture Organization's "1989 Country Tables: Basic Data on the Agricultural Sector." The cause of death comparisons were from the WHO annual statistics volume. The comparative medical systems information came from the *Statistical Abstracts of the United States* (1991), and used purchasing power parity which minimizes the gross distortions introduced by quoting dollar figures, which are heavily influenced by the balance of trade of each nation.

The analogy of the spacecraft to Mars was the author's, based on ideas from Alex Comfort's 1979 book.

2. A BATTLE JOINED

Nancy Donegan, Carol Ormes and John C. Rees were observed in action at Washington Hospital Center during March of 1991 through the good offices of James A. Curtain, the chief of medicine, and Claire Fiore, director of public affairs. The interchange about AIDS between the two Nobel laureates was reported by Richard Weiss in an excellent article about emerging viruses appearing in *Science Weekly.* Mortality data on recent infectious disease trends is from *Vital Statistics of the United States,* or the summaries published in *Monthly Vital Statistics Report* from the National Center for Health Statistics. For mortality from warfare see page 314 of Lancaster (1990) or see Garfield. Garfield notes World War II was the most lethal war, killing 3 percent of the world's population, an astounding loss. More detailed citations about the toll of infectious disease appear in the notes to chapters that follow. Details about the various pathogens in the medical environment, including CMV, were taken from the standard medical reference on the subject, Mandell (1990). More general properties of microscopic life-forms are described in Burnet (1975), Gould (1989) and Postgate (1986). For literature illustrating the difficulties of resistant *Staphylococcus aureus* in the hospital environment see Robert W. Haley, *Annals of Internal Medicine* (1982), 97:297, James E. Peacock, *Annals of Internal Medicine* (1980), 93:526, or Kent Crossley, *Journal of Infectious Disease* (1979), 139:280. An overview of the hospital battle with infectious disease appears in Nancy C. Griffith, *American Family Practice* (1987), 35:179. The story of the rabbit virus, myxomatosis, is told by many authors, and one treatment appears in Burnet (1975), page 137.

3. AFTER THE GARDEN OF EDEN

The very earliest history of man is mostly guesswork. This brief survey drew a little from many sources, including McNeill (1977), a landmark examination of the role of disease in human history; Chapter 1 in Lancaster (1990); and René Dubos, both *Mirage of Health* and a selection of Dubos's writing reprinted in Piel (1990), page 151. Another classic from earlier history is Zinsser (1935). The periods when man's earliest ancestors left the jungles, evolved on the savannahs and expanded over the globe change constantly as new evidence emerges. The figures were from Klein (1989).

The life expectancy figures for early man were drawn from Shigekazu Hishinuma's excellent paper, "Historical Review on the Longevity of the Human Beings." Hishinuma was the president of the Institute of Actuaries of Japan and delivered a lecture summarizing the results of his lifelong study in a 1976 lecture at an international meeting of actuaries in Tokyo. He also provided an accompanying paper. The copy of the paper used for this book was courtesy of the Society of Actuaries, Schaumburg, Illinois. Hishinuma's longevity estimates, as he explains in his paper, are generally much shorter than those of the standard references, notably Dubin (1949) and Acsádi-Nemeskéri (1970). Hishinuma makes the telling point that the longevity estimates of the earliest humans are based on burial sites that contain so few infant remains that they imply societies from primitive times to Rome had infant mortality rates lower than modern-day Sweden, one of the present leaders of the world. This seems highly unlikely. It is much more reasonable to assume many young infants and children simply weren't buried in ceremonial sites. He uses the bones to estimate adult life expectancy, but assumes infant mortality rates were comparable with primitive societies today, and therefore quite high. Hishinuma also offers the most thorough and systematic integration of many published sources. Much health literature still carries the strong flavor of Rousseau, and seems to imply that primitive humans were healthier before being corrupted by modern life. The only certain evidence on this controversy is the health surveys of the most primitive societies that still exist, for example, Buck (1968) and Buck (1970). There are also numerous studies of the Yanomamo Indians, the Maori, Australian aborigines, African Bushmen. None suggest any important variation from the age-old primitive pattern of high fertility and low life expectancy. Studies do exist showing that certain disorders, for example, the increase in blood pressure with advancing age, are not found in some primitive societies—for example, Lewis K. Dahl, *American Journal of Clinical Nutrition* (1972), 25:231. In others, coronary heart disease appears to be extremely rare, although the lack of modern medical facilities raises serious questions about the accurate identification of the disease. Diagnosing a heart attack requires serial blood tests and an electrocardiogram; for details see Hurst (1986), page 842. The Framingham study showed 23 percent of heart attacks were not diagnosed in even modern times. For details see James R. Margolis, *American Journal of Cardiology* (1973), 32:1. The key point, however, is that many variations in disease-specific mortality may be observed even when life expectancy or total mortality is similar or identical. There seems no evidence in the record to contradict the central fact that life expectancy in the advanced democracies has reached the highest point in the history of the species. The quote from Hippocrates is from the translation by Adams (1939).

The terrible toll of the plague is discussed in Braudel (1985), Chapter 1; Lancaster (1990), page 97; and McNeill, starting at page 132. An excellent feature on the plague is Charles L. Mee, Jr.'s, article in *Smithsonian*, February 1990, page 67. The biological consequences of the discovery of the new world are found in several sources, McNeill, page 176, and pages 35–36 in Braudel (1985). Florin (1971) discusses the devastation of the North American Indian population just before the English colonists arrived in Massachusetts.

Biographies of Edward Jenner can be found in Saunders (1982) and a chapter in Radetsky (1991). John Snow's contributions and his controversy over cholera came from J. P. Vandenbroucke, *Journal of Clinical Epidemiology* (1988), 41:1215; Bruce S. Schoenberg, *Mayo Clinic Proceed-*

ings (1974), 49:680; and Friedman (1989). An entire work on cholera, Pollizer (1959), also has an extensive historical section. A wonderful historical perspective on sanitation—which may overstate the achievements of reformers but eloquently attests to conditions at the time—was written in 1923 by C.E.A. Winslow. A charming popular summary can be found in Jay Stuller's article in the February 1991 *Smithsonian* magazine, page 126. A more academic approach is Duffy (1990).

There are uncounted works on the golden age of microbiology. My favorite is again René Dubos's life of Pasteur, Dubos (1950). Also see Krause (1981), Lechevalier (1965), the historical section on vaccines in Plotkin (1988), and for even more on Pasteur, Vallery-Radot (1937). Among the many sources on the discovery of antibiotic drugs are Hare (1970), Krause (1981), Sheehan (1982), Hobby (1985), Macfarlane (1979), Piel (1990) and a November 1990 *Smithsonian* magazine article by Edwin Kiester, Jr., page 173, "A curiosity turned into the first silver bullet against death."

4. THE GREAT LONGEVITY GAIN

For the story of the tremendous impact of tuberculosis, we return again to René Dubos. His book, *The White Plague,* republished in 1979 after many years out of print, was the primary source for the section on TB. Dubos also provided some of the background on pneumonia in Piel (1990), page 53.

Thomas McKeown is sometimes described as the first sociologist of medicine. His *Role of Medicine* became a landmark because he was one of the first to move beyond ritual self-congratulation over the great discoveries of microbiology and examine long-term mortality data systematically. His seminal discovery was the many-times-repeated pattern that the most terrifying diseases had already begun to decline before the means of medical control were devised. This pattern may well be repeated again with the AIDS virus. His other major work, *An Introduction to Social Medicine,* was sometimes quoted, and is well worth further study.

Samuel Preston's work shares with McKeown the great strength of being based on actual mortality data. His *Mortality Patterns in National Populations* (1976) is an important analysis, although it will be tough reading without a background in multivariate statistical analysis. In the great tradition of open scientific research, Preston also published the raw mortality data on which his analysis was based in *Life Tables for National Populations,* 1972. The analysis of nutrition was primarily my own, although John Allred of Ohio State University provided review and assistance. He also shared chapters of the upcoming book of which he is coauthor, Gallagher (in press). Sagan (1987) is also recommended reading for examination of the role of child care and infant mortality. My own analysis differs primarily from these excellent works in that I doubt a single "factor" explains the longevity gain. If a single influence exists, it is that stable and prosperous democracies empower individuals and groups to pursue a longer healthier life in ways too numerous to mention and almost impossible to measure.

5. GOD DOES PLAY DICE

Details of the meeting of the Vaccines and Related Biological Products Advisory Committee were taken from the transcript, available from the Food and Drug Administration public documents room. The years for which flu shortened life expectancy were assembled from several sources—1980 and 1988 from that year's Department of Health and Human Services publication, *Health in the United States.* The earlier pandemics were analyzed at an International Conference on Asian Influenza, reprinted as a separate supplement in *American Review of Respiratory Disease,* Volume 83. Also see the epidemiological section of Kilbourne (1987). Kilbourne's book is considered the major authority on influenza and was the source for most technical detail, along with Britain's major authority, Stuart-Harris (1985). Those who want a nontechnical explanation of the fundamentals of microbiology might see Renato Dulbecco's *Design of Life* (1987). For more on viruses, see Evans (1984). For a microbiology text, try Stryer (1988).

Alan Kendal's statement about lethal mutations was from an interview. Kendal is also author of an excellent summary of viral capabilities of influenza in a paper, *American Journal of Medicine* (1987), 83 (Suppl. 6A):4. The account of the flu epidemic of 1918 was taken from Crosby (1976) and Collier (1974). The quote from the young physician at Fort Devens was reported by N.R. Grist in the *British Medical Journal,* December 22, 1979, page 1632.

The spread of the 1957 influenza pandemic was analyzed in Pyle (1986); the United States effort to ramp up vaccine production and the experiences were described by William McLean at the International Conference. Kilbourne's description of the results of the 1957 effort to halt the epidemic was from an interview.

Two important documents trace the unfolding of the great swine flu episode. The participants in the earliest events in the crisis as it unfolded at Fort Dix reported their findings in great detail in a series of papers that make up a special supplement to the *Journal of Infectious Disease,* Volume 136, 1977. As noted in the text, the main events were ably reported in Neustadt (1978). This account, written by Neustad and Harvey Fineberg, is a classic case study and recommended to all students of the perils of national decision-making about infectious disease. A much briefer look appeared in Philip M. Boffrey, *Science* (1976), 192:636. Also, Kilbourne, Alan Kendal and Martin Goldfield were interviewed for this account. Those seeking a shorter, medically oriented overview of the whole subject may wish to review "Influenza Viruses," a chapter in Evans (1984), or the section at page 422 in Plotkin (1988). The material on the avian influenza outbreak was provided courtesy of the Department of Agriculture's Animal/Plant Health Inspection Service. Sources included "Avian Influenza in Pennsylvania: The Beginning," a manuscript by Robert J. Eckroad and Linda A. Silverman Bachman, and six issues of *Foreign Animal Disease Reports,* Numbers 12-3, 12-4, 13-1, 14-1, 14-2 and 14-3.

6. A VIRUS EMERGES

The events in Reston, Virginia, Zaire and Sudan were assembled primarily through interviews with Joseph McCormick, Peter B. Jahrling, Karl M. Johnson and Dan Dalgard. Many documents were also used, including the November 29, 1989, and December 5, 1989, statements from the United States Army Medical Research Institute of Infectious Disease. The most extensive newspaper accounts of the episode were written by Brett J. Blackledge of the Journal Newspapers in north suburban Virginia, which were supplemented by *Washington Post* reports written by D'Vera Cohn. The official version from the Centers for Disease Control appears in these issues of their publication, *Morbidity and Mortality Weekly Reports:* (1989), 38: 181; (1990), 39:22; (1990), 39:221. For contemporaneous scientific reporting also see Peter B. Jahrling, *Lancet* (1990), 1:502.

For an overview of the Ebola virus and related diseases see Karl M. Johnson's chapter in Evans (1984). The 1976 outbreak in Zaire was reported in *Journal of the World Health Organization* (1978), 56:271, with a listed author of "Report of an International Commission," but apparently written by Karl M. Johnson. Also see Pierre H. Sureau, *Review of Infectious Diseases* (1989), S790. McCormick reported his later findings that there were different strains in Sudan and Zaire in J. B. McCormick *Journal of Infectious Diseases* (1983), 147:264, and in Michael J. Buchmeir, *Journal of Infectious Diseases* (1983), 147:276, where McCormick was a coauthor. The remarkable fact that AIDS antibodies were detected in the stored serum samples collected in the 1976 Zaire episode was reported in Nzila Nzlambi, *NEJM* (1988), 318:276.

Those skeptical that chronic fatigue syndrome might be a figment of yuppie imagination might read the surgeon Thomas L. English's moving account of his own experiences in *JAMA* (1991), 265:964. The rare but remarkable side effects of Reye's syndrome, which apparently occurs when aspirin is given to children with chickenpox, are documented in Eugene S. Hurwitz, (1985), 313:849, and Karen M. Starko, *Pediatrics* (1980), 66:859. For more information on tryptophan, see Laurence Slutsker, *JAMA* (1990), 264:213; Leslie A. Swygert, *JAMA* (1990), 254:1698; and CDC's *Morbidity and Mortality Weekly Report* (1990), 39:589.

Those interested in more detailed analysis of emerging viruses should turn to the works of Stephen S. Morse of Rockefeller University. He is author of a brief summary in *Journal of Infectious Diseases* (1990), 162:1. A much more detailed version is a chapter in Fox (1991). Edwin D. Kilbourne considers the problem in *JAMA* (1991), 264:68, and Joshua Lederberg presents his views in *JAMA* (1988), 260:684.

7. RISE OF THE RISK FACTOR DISEASES

The estimates of how many American adults have high blood cholesterol were from Christopher Sempos, *JAMA* (1989), 262:45. The guidelines for the definition of high cholesterol are explained in the "Report of the Expert Panel on Detection, Evaluation, and Treatment of High Blood Cholesterol in Adults," National Cholesterol Education Program, National Heart, Lung, and Blood Institute, Bethesda, MD. The extent of high blood pressure is addressed in "Hypertension Prevalence and the Status of Awareness, Treatment, and Control in the United States," National High Blood Pressure Coordinating Committee, National Heart, Lung, and Blood Institute, Bethesda, MD. The prevalence of obesity was reported in "Health Implications of Obesity," National Institutes of Health Consensus Development Conference, reprinted in the *Annals of Internal Medicine* (1985), 103:983. The treatment with a 90 percent chance of failure is medically supervised diets to control obesity; they are examined at length in Chapter 8. The health advice that was not supported in five trials involves diet and heart disease and is discussed in Chapter 10, as is the clinical trial of a cholesterol-lowering drug in which 38 patients experienced side effects for each one who may have benefited.

The deaths attributable to coronary heart disease appear as Table 2 in "Excess Deaths from Nine Chronic Diseases in the United States, 1986," Robert A. Hahn, *JAMA* (1990), 264:2654. The deaths attributable to premature coronary heart disease—occurring at age 65 or before—were calculated by the author from Table 1-10 in *Vital Statistics of the United States, 1986*.

The facts and figures about the U.S. health system came from *Statistical Abstracts of the United States*. The employment comparisons were provided courtesy of the Employment Outlook staff, United States Department of Labor. The early incidence of appendicitis came from Dubin (1949); current losses were calculated from *Vital Statistics of the United States, 1987. Final Exit,* by Derek Humphry (1991) is identified in the bibliography.

The intention of targeting 25 percent of the adult population was disclosed in an interview by Basil M. Rifkind, chief, atherogenesis and lipid metabolism branch, National Heart, Lung, and Blood Institute. He described it as a purely arbitrary cutpoint for defining a high-risk population. The results actually achieved were reported in the Sempos article.

Marshall Becker's excellent article, "The Tyranny of Health Promotion," appeared in *Public Health Reviews* (1986), 14:15, and contains many other insights into health behaviors. Arthur J. Barsky's provocative essay "The Paradox of Health" appeared in *NEJM* (1988), 318:414.

The story of Joseph Goldberger's investigation of pellagra is a chapter in Gallagher. The possible infectious diseases Goldberger might have missed were included in training materials for the Centers for Disease

Control's Epidemiological Intelligence Service, which used Goldberger's landmark investigation as a case study.

The epidemiological missteps in the early studies of AIDS were analyzed by J. P. Vanderbrouche in the *American Journal of Epidemiology* (1989), 129:455. Examples he cited include "Risk Factors for Kaposi's Sarcoma in Homosexual Men," *Lancet* (1982), 1:1083, and a CDC task force report in *NEJM* (1982), 306:932. For a thoughtful examination of the problems of epidemiological studies see Alvan R. Feinstein's "Scientific Standards in Epidemiologic Studies of the Menace of Daily Life" in *Science* (1988), 242:1257.

The kind of evidence on smoking that existed in 1964 appears in the famous surgeon general's report, listed in the bibliography under Public Health Service. The later smoking intervention trials are examined in the Public Health Service's book *The Health Benefits of Smoking Cessation*, page 84.

8. OBESITY

Two overviews of obesity and its treatment are recommended for those who want to explore the issue on their own. Albert J. Stunkard of the University of Pennsylvania delivered two excellent lectures to the New York Academy of Medicine in December 1986, and they are reprinted in the *Bulletin of the New York Academy of Medicine* (1988), 64:903, 824. He also served as coeditor of the volume *Eating and Its Disorders,* an outstanding collection of papers drawing on the views of a diverse and interesting group of obesity researchers, which appears in the bibliography as Stunkard (1984). Susan C. Wooley of the University of Cincinnati is an eloquent proponent of the view that the extremely low success rate makes obesity treatment unwise in most instances. An example of her point of view appears in *Journal of the American Dietetic Association* (1991), 91:1248.

The primary source for the incidence of obesity is the Second National Health and Nutrition Examination Survey, 1976–80. However, an excellent summary appears in Lew (1990), pages 13–14 to 13–17. The arbitrary nature of this definition is discussed in the main text of Lew.

The size and scope of the commercial diet industry are outlined in

LaRosa (1989). He provided additional figures for the medically monitored programs in an interview.

The 1985 consensus conference on "The Health Implications of Obesity" appears as a special supplement to the *Annals of Internal Medicine* (1985), 103:978. It includes summaries of all 19 presentations and the final report.

The health risks of obesity are documented in the *Build Study, 1979,* cited in the bibliography as Society of Actuaries (1980). The actuarial risks were standardized and summarized in Lew (1990), at pages 13–38 to 13–48. The *Build Study* may slightly understate the risks of obesity for an additional reason—while it includes those who were insured, but medically impaired, it does not reflect those whose health status was so poor that no policy was issued at all.

The asthma guidelines, along with the drug company promotions, are identified in the bibliography under U.S. Department of Health and Human Services (1991). The edition mailed to at least some pediatricians included promotional letters from drug companies, which were omitted from those received directly from the National Heart, Lung, and Blood Institute.

George Blackburn's early experiments with liquid-protein diets were described by William J. Vitale, at page 630 of Subcommittee on Regulation, Business Opportunities and Energy (1990), Part II. The 60 deaths from the early liquid-protein diets are described in the AMA's Council on Scientific Affairs in *JAMA* (1988), 260:2547, and addressed by P. Felig, *NEJM* (1984), 310:589. Examples of the results of behavior modification weight loss may be found in F. Matthew Kramer, *International Journal of Obesity* (1989), 13:123. Thomas C. Wadden's promising results for combining behavior modification with a liquid-protein semistarvation diet were initially reported in *Journal of Consulting Clinical Psychiatry* (1986), 54:482. The program is reviewed in perspective by Albert J. Stunkard, *American Journal of Clinical Nutrition* (1987), 45:1142. In this article Stunkard also touted the "commercial opportunities" provided by this new treatment. The development of the Medifast program offered through physicians' offices was recounted by Vitale. The number of hospitals participating in the Optifast program was reported in testimony by William Rush, beginning at page 47, of Subcommittee on

Regulation, Business Opportunities and Energy (1990). This is the source for Lawrence Stifler's comments, although both Rush and Stifler were also interviewed.

The consulting relationships of Theodore Van Itallie, Thomas Wadden and George Blackburn were disclosed in a note to their article in *JAMA* (1990), 263:83. While some medical journals sometimes require disclosure of financial relationships, they are seldom disclosed as forthrightly as they were in this instance.

The study of 400 members of Kaiser Permanente health maintenance organization was published as Melbourne F. Hovell, *American Journal of Public Health* (1988), 78:663. The more optimistic characterization was from a Sandoz press kit on Optifast. Thomas J. Flynn was interviewed, and his letter can be found in *JAMA* (1990), 623:2885.

Oprah Winfrey revealed the positive side of rapid weight loss in a television show on December 15, 1988, and explored the "Pain of Regain" on November 5, 1990. The number of hospitals dropping the Optifast program was cited by William Rush in an interview. Medifast's fortunes were revealed in an interview with Janna Thornton, Medifast's director of program support. Optifast's Robert Hoerr was interviewed.

The long-term failure rate of obesity treatment is reported by Susan C. Wooley, in Stunkard (1984), and assessed in these articles: Teis Andersen, *International Journal of Obesity* (1988), L. E. Graham, *Journal of Consulting and Clinical Psychology* (1983), 51:322; and Thomas C. Wadden, *Journal of Consulting and Clinical Psychology* (1988), 56:925. C. Wayne Callaway was interviewed and wrote about the effects of semi-starvation in *Archives of Internal Medicine* (1989), 149:1750. Valerie Kirshy's story and Thomas Wadden's comment came from interviews.

9. HIGH BLOOD PRESSURE

A tape of the advertisement featuring the young man with dynamite strapped to his chest was provided courtesy of Citizens for Treatment of High Blood Pressure. Edward D. Freis's first effort to treat malignant hypertension was recalled in an interview, and described by him in a chapter about the origins and history of high blood pressure in Laragh (1990). The history and background also relied on Ackerknecht (1982) and Baldry (1971).

The risks of mild high blood pressure for a 45-year-old male were from The Blood Pressure Study, 1979; see Society of Actuaries (1980). The mortality rate differences were calculated from *Vital Statistics of the United States* for 1987. The talk on the incidence of malignant, severe, moderate, definite and mild high blood pressure was based on "Blood Pressure Levels in Persons 18–74 Years of Age in 1976–80," *Data from the National Health Survey,* Series 11, No. 234, National Center for Health Statistics, July 1986. The frequency of doctors' office visits for high blood pressure was reported in *Advance Data,* Number 209, April 28, 1992, National Center for Health Statistics, page 6, Table 9.

Edward D. Freis's two landmark clinical trials were reported as the Veterans Administration Cooperative Study Group on Antihypertensive Agents, *JAMA* (1967), 202:116, and *JAMA* (1970), 213:1143. The extraordinary career of Mary Lasker is described in Rettig (1978), and in the testimonial in *Gold Medal for Mary Lasker (H.R. 390),* Subcommittee on Consumer Affairs and Coinage (1987). Elliot Richardson's recollections were provided in an interview. Citizens for Treatment of High Blood Pressure's role in the crusade was described in part by its current executive director, Gerald Wilson. Merck's role was deduced by a copy of the actual manual used in the campaign and other materials.

These are the principal clinical trials of pharmacological interventions in hypertension:

Hypertension Detection and Follow-up (HDFP): Hypertension Detection and Follow-up Program Cooperative Group, *JAMA* (1979), 242:2562 and 242:2572; also *JAMA* (1982), 247:633, and *JAMA* (1988), 259:2113.
Australian Therapeutic Trial in Mild Hypertension: Report by the Management Committee, *The Lancet* (1980), 1:8181.
British MRC Trial: Medical Research Council Working Party, *British Medical Journal* (1985), 291:97.

For a review of all the trials considered together, see Jeffrey A. Cutler, *Hypertension* (1989), 13:I-36.

Rodney Jackson's comments about the risks and benefits of blood pressure treatment for women were from an interview. The HDFP results for women were examined in Peter L. Schnall, *New York State Journal of Medicine* (1984), 84:299.

Marshall Becker's comment was from an interview. Campbell

Moses's statement was made at a symposium reported in the *Annals of the New York Academy of Sciences* (1978), 304:84. Michael H. Alderman reviews the problem of labeling in *Journal of Clinical Epidemiology* (1990), 43:195. Side effects in the HDFP were reported in J. David Curb, *JAMA* (1985), 253:3263. For the British trial see Chapter 6 in Miall (1987). The quote about treating 850 patients to prevent one stroke was from the conclusions paragraph of the *British Medical Journal* report.

10. CHOLESTEROL

There are two overviews of the cholesterol literature that treat the cholesterol question in depth. One is my own earlier four-chapter treatment in Moore (1989); the current chapter tries to focus on new material. For the most comprehensive review in the scientific literature see Lars Werko's excellent analysis in *Acta Medica Scandinavica* (1987), 221:323. An overall examination of risk factor reduction and mortality appears in Robert M. Kaplan, *Medical Care* (1985), 23:5. A remarkably complete and objective review of a vast body of evidence that is so often distorted can be found in Toronto Working Group on Cholesterol Policy (1989).

The Finnish trial results are reported in Timo E. Strandberg, *JAMA* (1991), 266:1225. The accompanying editorial, "The Latest Report from Finland," appeared at page 1267. The excess mortality from clofibrate was a finding of M. F. Oliver, *British Heart Journal* (1978), 40:1069. The problems with the cholesterol-lowering thyroid hormone appeared in Coronary Drug Project Research Group, *JAMA* (1972), 220:996. The Merck grant to the American Medical Association to promote cholesterol treatment was first disclosed by Michael Waldholz in *The Wall Street Journal*, December 6, 1988, page B6.

The biological functions of the heart and the role of atherosclerosis in coronary heart disease are described in the cardiology text, Hurst (1986), a standard reference. The variability of cholesterol measurements is reported by D. M. Hegsted, *Proceedings of the National Academy of Science* (1987), 84:6260, and summarized by David Kritchevsky in Chapter 5 of Weininger (1985). Only a few autopsy studies have been performed to measure atherosclerosis in a population of otherwise healthy individuals. See *JAMA* (1983), 256:2683, and Duane M. Reed, *American Journal of Epidemiology* (1987), 126:214.

Beverly Teeters described her accidental acquisition of the consensus conference statement in an interview, and shared a copy of the document. The panel report appeared, without a named author other than "Consensus conference," in *JAMA* (1985), 253:2080. In 1981, the American Heart Association had outlined a cholesterol treatment program much like that eventually created—see Scott M. Grundy, *Circulation* (1982), 65:839A.

The grand strategy of the assault on coronary heart disease was described by one of those who helped shape it, George V. Mann of Vanderbilt University. He discussed the roots in a lecture to the Veritas Society on November 13, 1991. The basic epidemiological findings of Framingham are outlined in Dauber (1980). The lack of any link between life expectancy and cholesterol level after age 48 was reported by Keaven M. Anderson, *JAMA* (1987), 257:2176. The data presented show no relationship after age 48, but the abstract says after age 50. The 480,000 volunteers and screening criteria appear in "CPPT: Lipid Metabolism-Atherogenesis Branch, NHLBI, The Lipid Research Clinics Coronary Primary Prevention Trial Results," *JAMA* (1984), 251:251. The sad story of triparanol is told in Fine (1972). The fear of excess mortality from dextrothyroxine was reported by the Coronary Drug Project.

These are the major diet trials:

Veterans Administration: Seymour Dayton, *American Journal of Medicine* (1969), 46:751.
Minnesota Coronary Survey: Ivan D. Frantz, *Arteriosclerosis* (1989), 9:129.
MRFIT: Multiple Risk Factor Intervention Trial Research Group, *JAMA* (1982), 248:1465.
U.S. Heart-Diet cancellation is explained in *Arteriosclerosis: A Report by the National Heart, Lung, and Blood Institute Task Force on Arteriosclerosis,* June 1971, DHEW Pub. No. (NIH) 72-137.
WHO Multifactor: WHO European Collaborative Group, *European Heart Journal* (1983), 4:141.
Gothenburg: L. Wilhelmsen, *European Heart Journal* (1986), 7:279.
Oslo: I. Hjermann, *The Lancet* (1981), 2:1303.

The quote claiming diet is nonetheless the "cornerstone" of cholesterol-lowering treatment appears on page 36 of "Report of the Expert

Panel on Detection, Evaluation and Treatment of High Blood Cholesterol in Adults" (see Chapter 7 notes).

These are the drug trials cited:

WHO Clofibrate Trial: Oliver, M. F. *British Heart Journal* (1978), 40:1069.
Coronary Drug Project—niacin. Coronary Drug Project Research Group, *JAMA* (1975), 231:360.
Helsinki Heart Study: Frick, Heikki M., *NEJM* (1987), 317:1237.

Alan Brett's analysis appeared in *NEJM* (1989), 321:676. The statistics for cholesterol drugs actually prescribed were from Diane K. Wysowski, *JAMA* (1990), 263:2185.

The CLAS study, which examined the coronary arteries directly, was reported as David H. Blakenhorn, *JAMA* (1987), 257:3233. A four-year follow-up was published as Linda Cashin-Hemphill, *JAMA* (1990), 264:3013. The partial ileal bypass procedure results appeared as Henry Buchwald, *NEJM* (1990), 323:946.

The article about the fees that the medical experts charged drug companies was written by Teri Randall, and appeared in *JAMA* (1990), 264:1080. The episode involving Bernadine Healy, the director of NIH, was reported by Marilyn Chase in *The Wall Street Journal*, page 1, Jan. 26, 1989. The quote from the publication *It's YOUR Cholesterol* was from Volume 1, fall 1990, George Washington University Lipid Research Clinic. George Davey Smith and Juha Pekkanen's proposal for a moratorium on cholesterol drugs appeared in the *British Medical Journal* (1992), 304:431. Steven B. Hulley's editorial appeared in *Circulation* (1992), 86:1026.

11. WHAT'S IN YOUR GENES?

The fundamentals of genetics were taken from Chapter 5 in Wyngaarden (1992), Chapter 13 in Guyton (1987), Gardner (1991) and Thompson (1986).

Margaret H. Abbott's work with Raymond R. Pearl's famous collection of 2,319 nonagenarians was reported in M. R. Hawkins, *Bulletin of Hopkins Hospital* (1965), 117:24, and Margaret H. Abbott, *Hopkins Medical Journal* (1974), 134:1. The original Pearl book, which was not seen, was R. Pearl and R. Pearl, *The Ancestry of the Long-Lived,* Baltimore: The Johns Hopkins Press, 1944.

The Danish study of 960 adopted children appeared as Thorkild Sørensen, *NEJM* (1988), 318:727. The table showing family relationship and vulnerability to tuberculosis is from Burnet (1975), page 216. Albert Jacquard's assessment of the inheritability of longevity appeared as a chapter in Preston (1980); it was also the source for the longevity differences found in Danish twins. Another famous twins longevity study appears in the literature as F. S. Kallman, *Journal of Heredity* (1948), 39:349, *American Journal of Psychiatry* (1949), 106:29, and L. F. Jarvik, *American Journal of Human Genetics* (1960), 12:170.

The story of Huntington's disease, Duchenne's muscular dystrophy, retinoblastoma and cystic fibrosis came primarily from Bishop (1990), a book well worth exploring at length. Additional details are from Wyngaarden (1992). Familial hypercholesterolemia is described at page 574 in Hurst (1986). George Mann's comment on how this genetic disorder may have distorted the cholesterol-lowering trials was made at the Veritas Society meeting cited in the cholesterol chapter.

The possible longevity gene mutation that raises HDL levels was described in Akihiro Inazu, *NEJM* (1990), 323:1234, in Fumiko Saito, *Metabolism* (1984), 33:629, and in C. Glueck, *Journal of Laboratory and Clinical Medicine* (1976), 88:941.

The genetic predispositions and subsequent transformations resulting in colon cancer are described in a landmark sequence of papers in the same journal issue: Lisa A. Cannon, *NEJM* (1988), 319:533; Bert Vogelstein, at 319:524; and an editorial, Peter C. Nowell, at 319:575. The debate about a gene linked to alcoholism can be seen in K. Blum, *JAMA* (1990), 263:2055; Annabel M. Bolos, *JAMA* (1990), 264:3156; and Sandra J. Ackerman, *Journal of NIH Research* (1992), 4:61. The landmark study on inheritance of obesity was published as Albert J. Stunkard, *NEJM* (1986), 314:193.

There are many thoughtful discussions of the issues raised by our increasing knowledge of the human genome. Bishop (1990) explores it at some length, as do Holtzman (1989) and Arno G. Motulsky's analysis in *Science* (1983), 219:135.

12. LONGEVITY ADVANTAGES

The figures for marriage rates in the United States are from the Bureau of the Census (1990). Examples of the stress scale ratings of life events include Thomas H. Holmes, *Journal of Psychosomatic Research* (1967), 11:213, and Judith G. Rabkin, *Science* (1976), 194:1013. The historical studies of mortality and marriage are from Ellen Eliason Kisker, *Social Biology* (1987), 134:135, which also summarizes a vast body of other data. Another survey is Walter R. Grove, *American Journal of Sociology* (1972), 79:45. Marriage differentials also are found in Rogot (1988), which is referred to as a federal Mortality Study of One Million persons, and was a major reference for all the psychosocial indicators.

The Gothenburg, Sweden, study of mortality and marital status can be found in Annika Rosengren, *British Medical Journal* (1988), 297:1497. Mortality among the English nobility throughout several centuries was reported in a famous study, T. H. Hollingsworth, *Population Studies* (1957), 11:4. Mortality for the general population was from McKeown (1979). It is also discussed in Preston (1976). Mortality differences related to education are explored in Jacob J. Feldman, *American Journal of Epidemiology* (1989), 129:919.

The mortality study of military veterans discharged after World War II appears in *American Journal of Epidemiology* (1977), 105:559, and was also summarized in Lew (1990), pages 3-51.

One of the most detailed studies of Seventh-Day Adventists, and one that addresses the selection bias question directly, is Roland L. Phillips, *American Journal of Epidemiology* (1980), 112:296. Another study looks at Seventh-Day Adventist physicians and is reported in Daniel Ullmann, *JAMA* (1991), 265:2352. Mortality rates for the Baptist and other ministers were in Lew (1991), pages 3-62.

The figures for medical services to the poor and nonpoor population were presented by Gerry E. Hendershot, in *Health Affairs* (1988), spring issue, page 117. The actual data were from the Health Interview Survey, which the study's author supervised. To examine mortality in a poor black population, see the study of death rates in Harlem by Colin McCord, *NEJM* (1990), 322:173. The factors of race and social status are addressed in Vincente Navarro, in *The Lancet* (1990), 2:1238.

13. THE LIFESPAN OF CELLS AND OTHER CREATURES
Several books provide overviews of the biology of aging. A readable
primer is Arking (1991). The more difficult but classic work is Comfort
(1979). However, it is becoming dated in this fast-moving field. A
massive major work, especially strong in comparative animal studies, is
Finch (1990). For clarity and concise presentation in a difficult field, it
is hard to surpass Leonard Hayflick, who has written numerous articles
and chapter-length summaries, focusing mainly on aging at the cellular
level. For a broader summary, however, see Chapter 9 in Preston (1980)
and, for a cellular focus, page 21 in Warner (1987).

Thomas E. Johnson's nematode studies may be found in *Journal of
Gerontology* (1988), 4:B102, and *Science* (1990), 249:908. The other
animal comparisons are from Finch. The 28 markers for human aging
were in Shock (1984). The federal spending figures are from the federal
budget document, listed as Executive Office of the President (1990).
Richard Sprott's comments were from an interview.

The animal life strategies and contrasts were from Finch, with a few
examples from Comfort. The discussion about criteria for defining the
aging process appears in Arking (1991), page 8. He opts for a restrictive
definition requiring that true aging be a universal (rather than hetero-
geneous) process, but then is forced to make exceptions throughout the
book.

The studies of very long-lived humans include a section of Hayflick's
chapter in Preston (1980). The Vilcabamba episode is also told in R. B.
Mazess, *JAMA* (1978), 240:1781. For Georgians, see Zhores A. Medvedev, *Gerontologist* (1974), 14:381. A careful study of death rates around
age 100 can be found in Francisco R. Bayo, *Transactions of the Society of
Actuaries* (1983), 35:37, and John C. Wilkin, *Transactions of the Society of
Actuaries* (1981), 33:11.

Leonard Hayflick described his experiments in cell division in several
publications, including Warner (1987); *Experimental Gerontology* (1989),
24:355; *NEJM* (1976), 295:1302; *Scientific American* (1980), 242:58.

The new frontiers in aging research at the cellular level are summarized in great depth and detail in a special issue of *Mutation Research*
(1991), Volume 256. Calvin B. Hartley describes the possible role of
telomeres at page 271. The idea of abnormal cell growth as a fundamen-

tal concept of aging, as well as its possible role in coronary heart disease, was outlined by George Martin of the National Institute on Aging in an interview.

14. PRACTICAL LONGEVITY EXPERIMENTS

The diet-restriction experiments with monkeys were described by George S. Roth, of the Gerontology Research Center of the National Institute on Aging, in an interview. Additional details appear in Donald K. Ingram, *Journal of Gerontology* (1990), 45:B148, and in the monograph by Roth, appearing as Chapter 27 in Fishbein (1991).

Richard Weindruch's detailed experiment with mice is reported in *Journal of Nutrition* (1986), 116:641. For an overview of this increasingly complex field, see Edward J. Masoro, *Journal of Gerontology* (1988), 43:B56. He was also a coauthor of a study that seems to demonstrate that the effect of diet restriction is not simply to slow metabolism. It was published as R. McCarter, *American Journal of Physiology* (1985), 248:E488. The 1992 study of the effects of dieting on blood pressure in humans appeared as Trials of Hypertension Prevention Collaborative Research Group, *JAMA* (1992), 267:1213.

The literature on free radicals is so extensive that it will be only sampled here. An early but complete look at the subject can be found in Armstrong (1984). A brief but more recent conference summary is Carroll E. Cross, *Annals of Internal Medicine* (1987), 107:526. An even more recent and extensive look at free radicals appears as a special 1991 supplement to Volume 53 of the *American Journal of Clinical Nutrition*. Here a large selection of papers explore many of the questions, and most of the major figures in the field are represented. A critical, more skeptical analysis of the evidence appears in Martin Poot, *Mutation Research* (1991), 256:177. He makes many interesting objections. Hayflick is another skeptic, and his reservations may be seen in one of his summaries. William A. Pryor's model system was a chapter in Armstrong (1984). Winfred F. Malone was interviewed, and he also described the ongoing clinical trials in the *American Journal of Clinical Nutrition* (1991), 53:S305. The potential wonder drug, DHEA, is enthusiastically reviewed in depth by Arthur G. Schwartz in *Advances in Cancer Research* (1988), 51:391. Schwartz was also interviewed. The epidemiological study of DHEA and cardiovascular disease appeared in Elizabeth Barrett-

Connor, *NEJM* (1986), 315:1519. The potential effects on immune response were reported in Roger M. Loria, *Journal of Medical Virology* (1988), 26:301. The effects on memory were explored in James F. Flood, *Brain Research* (1988), 447:269. The two human studies of DHEA appeared in John E. Nestler, *Journal of Clinical Endocrinology and Metabolism* (1988), 68:57, and J. F. Mortola, *Journal of Clinical Endocrinology and Metabolism* (1990), 71:696. The widely reported growth hormone trial appeared in Daniel Rudman, *NEJM* (1990), 323:1, and an editorial by Mary Lee Vance at page 54 of the same issue.

15. SUMMING UP

The thoughts expressed in the final chapter were my own. The odds in the hypothetical lottery of life were calculated from a life table for the United States, 1988.

BIBLIOGRAPHY

Ackerknecht, Erwin A. *A Short History of Medicine*. Baltimore: Johns Hopkins University Press, 1982.

Adams, Francis, translator. *The Genuine Words of Hippocrates*. Baltimore: The Williams & Wilkins Company, 1939.

Arking, Robert. *Biology of Aging: Observations and Principles*. Englewood Cliffs, N.J.: Prentice-Hall, 1991.

Armstrong, Donald, R. S. Sohal, Richard G. Cutler, and Trevor F. Slater, editors. *Free Radicals in Molecular Biology, Aging, and Disease*. New York: Raven Press. 1984.

Baldry, P. E. *The Battle Against Heart Disease*. Boston: Cambridge University Press, 1971.

Berkman, Lisa F., and Lester Breslow. *Health and Ways of Living: the Alameda County Study*. New York: Oxford University Press, 1983.

Bishop, Jerry E., and Michael Waldholz. *Genome*. New York: Simon & Schuster, 1990.

Braudel, Fernand. *The Structures of Everyday Life*. New York: Harper & Row, Publishers, 1985.

Buck, Alfred A. *Health and Disease in Four Peruvian Villages, Contrasts in Epidemiology*. Baltimore: Johns Hopkins University Press, 1968.

Buck, Alfred A. *Health and Disease in Chad: Epidemiology, Culture and Environment in Five Villages*. Baltimore: Johns Hopkins University Press, 1970.

Bureau of the Census. *Statistical Abstract of the United States 1991*. Washington, D.C.: U.S. Department of Commerce, 1990.

Bureau of the Census. *World Population Profile: 1989*. Washington, D.C.: U.S. Department of Commerce, 1989.

Burnet, MacFarlane, and David O. White. *Natural History of Infectious Disease*. Cambridge, England: Cambridge University Press, 1975.

Carpenter, Kenneth J. *The History of Scurvy & Vitamin C*. Cambridge, England: Cambridge University Press, 1986.

Collier, Richard. *The Plague of the Spanish Lady*. New York: Atheneum, 1974.

Comfort, Alex. *The Biology of Senescence*. New York: Elsevier, 1979.

Cousins, Norman. *Head First: The Biology of Hope*. New York: E. P. Dutton, 1989.

Crosby, Alfred W., Jr. *Epidemic and Peace, 1918*. Westport, Connecticut: Greenwood Press, 1976.

Dauber, Thomas Royle. *The Framingham Study*. Cambridge, Mass.: Harvard University Press, 1980.

Dawkins, Richard. *The Blind Watchmaker*. New York: W. W. Norton & Company, 1987.

Delaporte, Francois. *Disease and Civilization*. Cambridge, Mass.: The MIT Press, 1986.

Delgadillo, Linda M., editor. *The Future of Life Expectancy*. Schaumberg, Ill.: Society of Actuaries, 1980.

Dubin, Louis I., Alfred J. Lotka, and Mortimer Spiegelman. *Length of Life*. New York: The Ronald Press Company, 1949.

Dubos, René J. *Louis Pasteur: Free Lance of Science*. Boston: Little, Brown & Company, 1950.

Dubos, René. *The Mirage of Health*. New York: Harper & Row, 1959. Perennial Library Edition.

Dubos, René. *The White Plague*. New Brunswick, N.J.: Rutgers University Press, 1979.

Duffy, John. *The Sanitarians*. Urbana, Ill.: The University of Illinois Press, 1990.

Dulbecco, Renato. *The Design of Life*. New Haven, Conn.: Yale University Press, 1987.

Duncan, Ronald, and Miranda Weston-Smith. *The Encyclopedia of Medical Ignorance*. Oxford, England: Pergamon Press, Ltd., 1984.

Evans, Alfred S., editor. *Viral Infections of Humans*. New York: Plenum Medical Book Company, 1984.

Executive Office of the President. *Budget of the United States Government Fiscal Year 1991*. Washington, D.C.: U.S. Government Printing Office, 1990.

Finch, Caleb E. *Longevity, Senescence, and the Genome*. Chicago: University of Chicago Press, 1990.

Fine, Ralph Adam. *The Great Drug Deception.* New York: Stein and Day, 1972.

Fishbein, L., editor. *Biological Effects of Dietary Restriction.* Berlin: Springer-Verlag, 1991.

Florin, John W. *Death in New England.* Chapel Hill, N.C.: University of North Carolina, 1971.

Fox, D. M., and E. Fee. *AIDS: Contemporary History.* Berkeley: University of California Press, 1991.

Friedman, David A. *Statistical Models and Shoe Leather.* Berkeley: University of California Statistics Department, Technical Report No. 217, 1989.

Fuchs. Victor R. *Who Shall Live?* New York: Basic Books, 1974.

Gallagher, Charlotte, and John Allred. *Taking the Fear Out of Eating.* New York: Cambridge University Press, (in press).

Gardner, Eldon John. *Principles of Genetics.* New York: John Wiley & Sons, 1991.

Gould, James L., and Carol Grant Gould, editors. *Life at the Edge: Readings from Scientific American Magazine.* New York: W. H. Freeman and Company, 1989.

Guyton, Arthur C. *Human Physiology and Mechanisms of Disease.* Philadelphia: W. B. Saunders Company, 1987.

Halliwell, Barry, and John M. C. Gutteridge. *Free Radicals in Biology and Medicine,* 2nd ed. Oxford: Oxford University Press, 1989.

Hare, Ronald. *The Birth of Penicillin.* London: George Allen and Unwin, Ltd.: 1970.

Hobby, Gladys L. *Penicillin: Meeting the Challenge.* New Haven: Yale University Press, 1985.

Holtzman, Neil A. *Proceed with Caution: Predicting Genetic Risks in the Recombinant DNA Era.* Baltimore: Johns Hopkins University Press, 1989.

Humphry, Derek. *Final Exit: The Practicalities of Self-Deliverance & Assisted Suicide for the Dying.* New York: Carol Publishing, 1991.

Hurst, J. Willis, editor-in-chief. *The Heart,* 6th ed. New York: McGraw-Hill Book Company, 1986.

Hustead, Edwin C., *100 Years of Mortality.* Schaumberg, Ill.: Society of Actuaries, 1989.

Ibrahim, Michel A. *Epidemiology and Health Policy.* Rockville, Maryland: Aspen Systems Corporation, 1985. RA 652.4.127.

Illich, Ivan. *Medical Nemesis.* New York: Pantheon Books, 1976.

Jensen, Marcus M., and Donald N. Wright. *Introduction to Microbiology.* Englewood Cliffs, N.J.: Prentice-Hall, 1989.

Kaplan, Norman M. *Clinical Hypertension,* 5th ed. Baltimore: Williams & Wilkins, 1990.

Kendal, Alan P., and Peter A. Patriarca, editors. *Options for the Control of Influenza.* New York: Alan R. Liss, Inc., 1986.

Kilbourne, Edwin D. *Influenza.* New York: Plenum Medical Book Company, 1987.

Klein, Richard. *The Human Career: Human Biological and Cultural Origins.* Chicago: University of Chicago Press, 1989.

Krause, Richard M. *The Restless Tide.* Washington, D.C.: National Foundation for Infectious Diseases, 1981.

Lancaster, H. O. *Expectations of Life: A Study in the Demography, Statistics, and History of World Mortality.* New York: Springer-Verlag, 1990.

Laragh, J. J., and B. M. Brenner, editors. *Hypertension: Pathophysiology, Diagnosis, and Management.* New York: Raven Press, Ltd., 1990.

LaRosa, John. *Weight Loss & Diet Control Market.* Valley Stream, N.Y.: Marketdata Enterprises, Inc., 1989.

Lechevalier, Hubert A., and Morris Solotorovsky. *Three Centuries of Microbiology.* New York: McGraw-Hill Book Company, 1965.

Lew, Edward A., and Jerzy Gajewski, editors. *Medical Risks: Trends in Mortality and Time Elapsed,* 2 vols. New York: Praeger Publishers, 1990.

Lonergan, Edmund T., II, editor. *Extending Life, Enhancing Life: A National Research Agenda on Aging.* Washington, D.C.: National Academy of Sciences, 1991.

Macflarlane, Gwyn. *Howard Florey: The Making of a Great Scientist.* New York: Oxford University Press, 1979.

Mandell, Gerald L., R. Gordon Douglas, Jr., and John E. Bennett, editors. *Principles and Practice of Infectious Diseases,* 3rd ed. New York: Churchill Livingstone, 1990.

Marks, Geoffrey, and William K. Beatty. *Epidemics.* New York: Charles Scribner's Sons, 1976.

McKeown, Thomas. *The Role of Medicine.* Princeton, N.J.: Princeton University Press, 1979.

McKeown, Thomas, and C. R. Lowe. *An Introduction to Social Medicine.* Oxford, England: Blackwell Scientific Publications, 1974.

McKusick, Victor A. *Mendelian Inheritance in Man.* Baltimore: Johns Hopkins University Press, 1988.

McNeill, William H. *Plagues & Peoples.* New York: Doubleday Anchor Books, 1977.

Meyer, John A. *Lung Cancer Chronicles.* New Brunswick, N.J.: Rutgers University Press, 1990.

Miall, W. E., and Gillian Greenberg. *Mild Hypertension: Is There Pressure to Treat?* Cambridge: Cambridge University Press, 1987.

Moore, Thomas J. *Heart Failure: A Critical Inquiry into American Medicine and the Revolution in Coronary Care.* New York: Random House, 1989.

National Center for Health Statistics. *Obese and Overweight Adults in the United States.* Series 11, No. 230. National Center for Health Statistics, Hyattsville, Maryland. 1983.

National Institutes of Health. *Obesity in America.* Washington, D.C.: United States Public Health Service, 1979.

Neustadt, Richard E., and Harvey V. Fineberg. *The Swine Flu Affair.* Washington D.C.: U.S. Department of Health, Education and Welfare, 1978.

Payer, Lynn. *Medicine & Culture.* New York: Henry Holt & Company, 1988.

Pearson, Durk, and Sandy Shaw. *Life Extension: A Practical Scientific Approach.* New York: Warner Books, 1983.

Pickering, George White. *High Blood Pressure.* London: Churchill, 1968.

Piel Gerard, editor. *The World of René Dubos.* New York: Henry Holt and Company, 1990.

Plotkin, Stanley A., and Edward A. Mortimer. *Vaccines.* Philadelphia: W. B. Saunders Company, 1988.

Pollizer, R. *Cholera.* Geneva: World Health Organization, 1959.

Postgate, John. *Microbes and Man.* Middlesex, England: Penguin Books, Ltd., 1986.

Preston, Samuel H. *Mortality Patterns in National Populations.* New York: Academic Press, 1976.

Preston, Samuel H., editor. *Biological and Social Aspects of Mortality and the Length of Life.* Liege, Belgium: Ordina Editions, 1980.

Preston, Samuel H., Nathan Keyfitz, and Robert Shoen. *Causes of Death: Life Tables for National Populations.* New York: Seminar Press, 1972.

Public Health Service. *Smoking and Health: Report of the Advisory Committee to the Surgeon General of the Public Health Service.* Washington, D.C.: U.S. Government Printing Office, 1964.

Public Health Service. *Healthy People: The Surgeon General's Report on Health Promotion and Disease Prevention.* Washington, D.C.: U.S. Department of Health, Education and Welfare, 1979.

Public Health Service, Office on Smoking and Health. *Reducing the Health Consequences of Smoking: 25 Years of Progress.* Rockville, Maryland: Centers for Disease Control, 1989.

Public Health Service, Office on Smoking and Health. *The Health Benefits of Smoking Cessation. A Report of the Surgeon General.* Rockville, Maryland: Centers for Disease Control, 1990.

Public Health Service. *Prevention '89/90: Federal Programs and Progress.* Washington, D.C.: U.S. Department of Health and Human Services, 1990.

Pyle, Gerald F. *The Diffusion of Influenza.* Totawa, N.J.: Rowman & Littlefield, 1986.

Radetsky, Peter. *The Invisible Invaders: The Story of the Emerging Age of Viruses.* Boston: Little, Brown & Company, 1991.

Rettig, Richard A. *Cancer Crusade: the Story of the National Cancer Act of 1971.* Princeton, N.J.: Princeton University Press, 1978.

Rogot, Eugene, et al. *A Mortality Study of One Million Persons.* Bethesda, Md.: National Institutes of Health, 1988.

Roitt, Ivan M., Jonathan Brostoff, and David K. Male. *Immunology.* London, England: Gower Medical Publishing, 1989.

Sagan, Leonard A. *The Health of Nations.* New York: Basic Books, 1987.

Saunders, Paul. *Edward Jenner: The Cheltenham Years.* Hanover, N.H.: University Press of New England, 1982.

Sheehan, John C. *The Enchanted Ring: The Untold Story of Penicillin.* Cambridge, Mass.: MIT Press, 1982.

Shock, Nathan. *Normal Human Aging: The Baltimore Longitudinal Study of Aging.* NIH Publication No. 84-2450. Bethesda, Md.: National Institutes of Health, 1984.

Siegel, Bernie S. *Love, Medicine & Miracles.* New York: Harper & Row, 1988.

Snell, Richard S. *Atlas of Clinical Anatomy.* Boston: Little, Brown & Company, 1978.

Society of Actuaries and Association of Life Insurance Medical Directors. *Blood Pressure Study, 1979.* Schaumberg, Ill.: Society of Actuaries, 1980.

Society of Actuaries and Association of Life Insurance Medical Directors. *Build Study, 1979.* Schaumberg, Ill.: Society of Actuaries, 1980.

Starr, Paul. *The Social Transformation of American Medicine.* New York: Basic Books, 1982.

Stryer, Lubert. *The Molecular Design of Life.* New York: W. H. Freeman Company, 1988.

Stuart-Harris, Charles H., Geoffrey C. Schild, and John S. Oxford. *Influenza: The Viruses and the Disease.* London: Edward Arnold, Ltd., 1985.

Stunkard, A. J., and E. Stellar. *Eating and Its Disorders.* New York: Raven Press, 1984.

Subcommittee on Consumer Affairs and Coinage, Committee on Banking, Finance and Urban Affairs, House of Representatives. *Gold Medal for*

Mary Lasker (H.R. 390), September 15, 1987. Washington, D.C.: U.S. Government Printing Office, 1987.

Subcommittee on Regulation, Business Opportunities and Energy, Committee on Small Business. *Deception and Fraud in the Diet Industry,* Parts I & II. Washington, D.C.: U.S. Government Printing Office, 1990.

Thomas, Lewis. *The Youngest Science.* New York: The Viking Press, 1983.

Thompson, James S., and Margaret W. Thompson. *Genetics in Medicine.* Philadelphia: W. B. Saunders Company, 1986.

Toronto Working Group on Cholesterol Policy. *Detection and Management of Asymptomatic Hypercholesterolemia.* Toronto: Ontario Ministry of Health, 1989.

Trowbridge, Charles L. *Fundamental Concepts of Actuarial Science.* Schaumberg, Ill.: Actuarial Education and Research Fund, 1989.

U.S. Department of Commerce. *Vital Statistics Rates in the United States 1900–1940.* Washington, D.C.: Government Printing Office, 1943.

U.S. Department of Health and Human Services. *A Report of the Expert Panel on Detection, Evaluation and Treatment of High Blood Cholesterol in Adults.* Washington, D.C.: Public Health Service, National Institutes of Health, 1988.

U.S. Department of Health and Human Services. *Guidelines for the Diagnosis and Management of Asthma.* Washington, D.C.: Public Health Service, National Institutes of Health, 1991.

Vallery-Radot, Rene. *The Life of Pasteur.* New York: The Sun Dial Press, Inc., 1937.

Warner, H. R., editor. *Modern Biological Theories of Aging.* New York: Raven Press, 1987.

Weininger, Jean, and George M. Briggs. *Nutrition Update,* Volume 8. New York: John Wiley & Sons, 1985.

Winslow, C.E.A. *Evolution and Significance of the Modern Public Health Campaign.* New Haven: Yale University Press, 1923.

World Health Organization. *Levels and Trend of Mortality Since 1950.* New York: United Nations, 1982.

World Health Organization. *World Health Statistics Annual.* Geneva, Switzerland: World Health Organization, 1989.

Wyngaarden, James B., Lloyd H. Smoth, and J. Claude Bennett. *Cecil Textbook of Medicine.* Philadelphia: W. B. Saunders Company, 1992.

Zinsser, Hans. *Rats, Lice and History.* New York: Blue Ribbon Books, Inc., 1935.

INDEX